pocket guide to

ESSENTIAL OILS

the mindful living guides

— pocket guide to —

ESSENTIAL OILS

USING AROMATHERAPY
FOR HEALTH & HEALING

Previously published as
Pocket Guide to Aromatherapy

KATHI KEVILLE

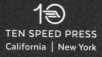

TEN SPEED PRESS
California | New York

I dedicate this book to everyone who has ever smelled a flower, sniffed the first scent of spring in the air, or walked down the fragrant path of an herb garden. May your lives always be filled with fragrance!

Thank you to all the modern pioneers of aromatherapy who have brought this ancient art to the attention of the world. Thank you especially to aromatherapist Mindy Green, my friend and coauthor of *Aromatherapy: A Complete Guide to the Healing Art*. Her knowledge and inspiration are reflected in this pocket guide.

CONTENTS

WHAT ARE
ESSENTIAL OILS?

Essential oils are potent aromatic substances extracted from fragrant plants for physical and emotional healing. Today, herbalists, body workers, cosmetologists, chiropractors, and other holistic healers are discovering how using these oils in a multifaceted and versatile healing art called aromatherapy can enrich their practices. You can use the same principles of aromatherapy as a natural remedy in your home.

Interest in therapeutic essential oils continues to grow. They are pumped into offices, stores, and even some hospitals to make the atmosphere more relaxing. Large corporations are turning to fragrance to keep their workers alert and more content on the job now that certain scents have been shown to lower blood pressure, relieve anxiety, and improve mental focus.

There are many approaches to using essential oils. Applied externally, they penetrate through the skin into underlying tissues to reach the bloodstream: compounds from lavender oil have been detected in the blood only twenty minutes after it was rubbed on the skin. As a result, one can treat a wide range of physical conditions using essential oils. For example, rubbing an aromatic vapor balm containing eucalyptus on the chest relieves lung congestion and fights infection through inhalation deep into air passages and also through absorption of the oils into the chest.

The beauty of essential oils is that you can take advantage of both their physical and emotional effects in the same treatment. A chamomile body oil massaged on the abdomen to soothe indigestion can also calm nervous conditions. A body lotion that improves your complexion can also contain essential oils that relieve depression.

In this book, I describe these methods, providing recipes along the way to get you started with essential oils. For even more detail about using essential oils and making your own products, look for *Aromatherapy: A Complete Guide to the Healing Art*.

QUESTIONS MOST FREQUENTLY ASKED ABOUT ESSENTIAL OILS

With today's growing emphasis on natural solutions to mind and body issues, more and more people are curious about aromatherapy and essential oils. The following are answers to questions I often hear.

Is Aromatherapy a New Science?

The use of aromatic herbs in aromatherapy dates back to at least 4000 BCE, when Neolithic people made ointments by combining fat and aromatic plants. Throughout the world, cultures used aromatic steams, smoke, and waters for healing long before essential oils were extracted from plants. Around 3000 BCE, the uses of odoriferous herbs were recorded on papyrus in Egypt and on clay tablets in Mesopotamia and Babylonia. By 1700 BCE, trade routes had been established throughout the Middle East, in part to traffic solid aromatic unguents; myrrh and frankincense for incense, perfume, and medicine; and aromatic spices for food. The routes extended into India, China, and Europe.

Primitive distillers may have produced fragrant waters as early as 500 CE. In the eleventh century, distillers became sophisticated enough to produce quantities of pure essential oil.

Modern aromatherapy was born when René-Maurice Gattefossé, a French chemist descended from a long line of perfumers, reunited perfumery and medicine. He coined the term *aromatherapy* around 1928 following an accident in his family's perfume factory. When a laboratory explosion severely burned his hand, he plunged it into a container of lavender essential oil and was amazed at how quickly the burn healed. Young Gattefossé began to look for an answer. His writings inspired others to explore the use of essential oils for medicinal purposes.

How Is Aromatherapy Connected to Herbalism?

Herbalism is the use of herbs and herbal preparations to treat medicinal conditions and to maintain health. Throughout the world, aromatherapy always has been a part of herbalism. If you have ever enjoyed an herbal tea or used lotion scented with herbs, then you have already experienced aromatherapy. When you make a tea—say peppermint or chamomile—the heat draws essential oils from the plant into the water. You receive the healing properties both as you drink the tea and as you inhale the aroma.

Aromatherapy differs from herbalism because it employs only *fragrant* herbs. I think of it as a branch of herbalism, but one that uses fragrant plants exclusively. The aromatic essential oils found in all fragrant plants give them their scent and contribute to their medicinal properties. Some herbs contain these oils and some do not. Aromatic thyme, ginger, and myrrh are used in both aromatherapy and herbalism. Nonfragrant herbs such as comfrey or goldenseal are found only in herbalism. There are also a few plants that produce therapeutic essential oils commonly used in aromatherapy, such as ylang-ylang and helichrysum, that herbalists seldom use. Because the essential oil is typically only one among a wider spectrum of medicinal compounds found in an herb, herb books describing a fragrant herb's properties may not always be referring to the properties in the essential oil.

Why Are Essential Oils Fragrant?

Essential oils consist of tiny aromatic molecules that are released from a fragrant plant when it's crushed or that escape into the air during the heat of the day. This is what makes herb gardens so fragrant! Essential oils are composed of many different aromatic molecules—more than thirty thousand have been identified and named. A single essential oil can contain more than one hundred different types of these molecules, with each one contributing its own aroma and medicinal use. Essential oils are like puzzles with their fragrance and actions determined by which aromatic pieces they contain.

A vast number of possible combinations of fragrant molecules is needed to produce so many unique plant fragrances. Our sense of smell is keen enough to differentiate one from the other. As you sniff your way through a selection of essential oils, you'll notice that some have similar scents. That is because the same fragrant molecules can occur in more than one plant, even when the plants are unrelated. This is true of plants that produce a lemonlike aroma; they include lemon verbena, melissa (lemon balm), lemon thyme, lemon eucalyptus, citronella, palmarosa, and lemon itself. All of these plants and their corresponding essential oils smell lemony, yet each one possesses a slightly different combination of aromatic molecules that carries its own distinctive olfactory shading. In a few cases, a plant's essential oil is composed chiefly of one type of molecule and scent. For example, sandalwood contains up to 90 percent santalol, and clove bud has between 70 percent and 80 percent eugenol.

Why Are There Different Names for the Same Oil?

Botany organizes plants according to how closely they visually resemble each other. These families are grouped into individual genera, which are then identified as individual species. There is sometimes also a subspecies. For example, lavender is in the mint family under the genus *Lavandula*. The species most commonly used as essential oil are either *Lavandula angustifolia* or a hybrid version, *Lavandula × intermedia*. The essential oil from the hybrid is less expensive because the plant is easier to grow and produces more flowers that contain a greater quantity of oil.

Each of the many other lavender species has its own distinguishing flower and scent. Therapeutic properties may vary among species. *Lavandula spicta* contains more camphor compounds, giving it a harsher smell but making it even more suitable to put into a liniment. Other essential oil–bearing plants in which multiple species are commonly distilled into essential oil include basil, cedarwood, chamomile, eucalyptus, lavender, oregano, sage, tea tree, and thyme.

Sometimes botanists further divide species into a subspecies or variety, often designated as "var." A variety that has been created through cultivation techniques is called a cultivar in the plant nursery trade. There are hundreds of lavenders, although only a few are distilled for commercial sale. Examples of lavender cultivars sold in plant nurseries are *Lavandula × intermedia* 'Grosso' and 'Hidcote'. In this book, you will find discussion of a bitter orange variety, *Citrus aurantium* var. *amara*. Some aromatherapists may seek out a particular species because it is known to be effective—for instance, the tea tree species named niaouli (*Melaleuca quinquenervia*) for its particularly potent antiviral properties.

It is the most transparent when labels on products and descriptive brochures provide each essential oil's full botanical name to avoid confusion. Sometimes, the same common name is used for more than one plant. Cedarwood can actually refer to quite a few essential oils that are derived from plants that are not even in the same genus. Many essential oils also have several common names. For example, helichrysum is also known as immortale and curry plant.

What Is an Essential Oil Chemotype?

Chemists use the term *chemotype* to designate a plant that has slightly different chemistry from others in the same species, even though botanists view them as the same plant. The quantity of individual compounds in a chemotype essential oil usually varies from the original plant. This alters the overall smell and properties. Growing conditions can change the percentages of aromatic compounds. Once a plant is adapted to a new area, it may retain its new chemotype even when transplanted somewhere else. Not all plants easily morph into chemotypes, but rosemary and thyme are good examples of essential oils that do. Aromatherapists may seek a particular chemotype; for instance, rosemary *(Rosmarinus officinalis* ct. *verbenone)* is sought out because it is particularly good in treating sinus infection, muscle spasms, and oily skin.

Why Do Plants Produce Essential Oils?

At first, botanists didn't understand why plants bother to create essential oils, which seemed to be mere by-products of plant metabolism. Botanical research has discovered that essential oils serve important functions that contribute to plant health. Fragrance attracts insects that fertilize flowers while repelling destructive insects and other predators from eating the plant. Many aromatic plants increase their scent production when something takes a bite of them. This makes them less tasty and may even serve as an aromatic distress signal that is relayed from one plant to another. In addition, *terpene* compounds help waterproof the plant to protect it from rain. Most essential oils are antiseptic, preventing the growth of bacteria, mold, and fungus on a plant.

How Are Essential Oils Obtained from Plants?

Essential oils are most often extracted from plants through *steam distillation*. Fresh or dried plant material is suspended over boiling water inside a closed container. As the hot steam from the water rises, it easily pulls the tiny essential oil compounds out of the plant. The next step rapidly cools the steam back into water. During this cooldown, the essential oil separates from the water. Called a *hydrosol*, the resulting water often retains the most water-soluble fractions of the essential oil, making it fragrant. Since it carries only part of the essential oil, it may not have all the healing properties of the whole oil. The essential oils in some flowers, such as carnation, violet, and gardenia, are too fragile to endure the heat produced during steam distillation. These oils are usually available only as synthetics.

There are several other ways to produce essential oils. Citrus peels can be pressed to release their essential oil. An old method, rarely used today, is *enfleurage*, which extracts the oils into sheets of warm fat. Chemical solvents are also used to extract essential oils, and then the often toxic solvent is removed. The resulting oil is called an *absolute*. A new method (albeit an expensive one) extracts oil using carbon dioxide. These CO_2-extracted essential oils carry a scent that smells the closest to the original plant because this process does not use heat.

Can I Make My Own Essential Oils?

You can indeed make essential oils at home—but do not expect to produce much! Distillation demands a large supply of plant material. Only a small vial of essential oils results from a wheelbarrow full of plants. The oil can be distilled from either fresh or dried plant material. Fresh plants contain about 30 percent more essential oil than dried plants. On the other hand, distilling dried plants means that much more plant material fits in the distiller.

You can purchase your own steam distiller. A tabletop distiller designed to hold a gallon or less of plant material mostly produces hydrosols—the scented water resulting from distillation—with perhaps a few drops of essential oil, depending upon which plant is being distilled. Larger, more expensive distillers produce essential oil as well as hydrosol.

You can also obtain some hydrosol by rigging up kitchen pots. Place water in a pan that has aromatic plants in a steamer held above it—just as you would steam vegetables, but with aromatic herbs instead. Balance a bowl inside the pan on top of the plant material. Turn the pan's lid upside down on the top of the pan and fill it with ice. Put the pan on a stove burner and turn the heat to medium high. As the water boils, steam will rise through the plant material and pick up its essential oils. The ice-cold lid will cool the fragrant steam, which then falls down and collects in the bowl as aromatic water.

Why Are Some Essential Oils So Much More Expensive Than Others?

The broad price range of essential oils—from six to one thousand dollars per ounce—reflects the difficulty involved in cultivating, collecting, producing, and storing different types. It is no wonder that Bulgarian rose essential oil is so expensive when you consider that it takes about six hundred pounds of rose petals to produce one ounce! Plus, rose bushes are high maintenance since they must be carefully cultivated, pruned, and hand-harvested. On the other hand, plants such as eucalyptus and rosemary are easy to grow and yield a comparatively large amount of essential oil, placing them among the least expensive oils.

What About Sustainability?

We live in a world where environmental change and product demand are taking a toll on natural resources. Essential oils are no exception. Problems with sustainability occur with plants harvested from the wild. The United Plant Savers organization (unitedplantsavers.org) and the Convention on International Trade in Endangered Species (CITES) have both investigated the harvest of aromatic plants. Trees are the most problematic since they are generally cut down to distill. The only plantation-grown sandalwood essential oil is coming from Australia. Bois de rose *(Aniba rosaeodora)* oil has a lovely scent, but these trees only grow in wild Amazon jungles where they are cut down for their essential oil. It is difficult to find, but a small amount of very expensive bois de rose is said to be harvested from just the small branches of standing trees. There are other overharvested trees that are currently cut down from the wild. Try to find sustainable sources of Indian myrrh *(Commiphora wightii)*, Atlas cedarwood *(Cedrus abrahamii)*, silver fir *(Abies alba)*, agarwood *(Aquilaria rostrate)*, and frankincense *(Boswellia spp.)* and the related, palo santo *(Bursea graveolens)*. Some herbaceous plants are also in danger of extinction. Purchase spikenard or jatamansi *(Nardostachys gradiflota)* essential oil that is cultivated in Nepal rather than harvested from the wild.

Many plants used for essential oil production are cultivated in economically poor countries. This keeps down the price of essential oils, but many farmers are paid low wages and their livelihood depends upon their crop. Besides supporting farmers, cultivated essential oils do not use more cropland than the corresponding herbs. That is because essential oil is usually diluted down to 1 or 2 percent before using it—an amount just a little stronger than what we find in the plant. The result is that often roughly the same amount of acreage is used whether the crop goes to herbs or essential oil.

How Does Fragrance Affect Emotions?

When your olfactory sensors detect a particular aroma, this information is sent to the brain's primitive limbic system and then areas that influence memory, learning, emotions, hormone balance, and basic survival mechanisms, such as the fight-or-flight response. Researchers studying the science of medicinal aromas discovered that exposure to aromatic substances alters brain waves and reactions. The fragrance research company International Fragrance and Flavor (IFF) tested more than two thousand subjects to show that scent relieves pain, calls up deep-seated memories, and affects personality, behavior, and sleep patterns by how they affect the brain. Aroma is assisting truck drivers, railroad engineers, air traffic controllers, and others whose jobs require that they remain alert.

Why Are So Many Cosmetologists Working with Essential Oils?

Major cosmetics firms, such as Avon, Revlon, and Japan's Shiseido discovered in their labs that essential oils offer a complete health and beauty package for both skin and hair care. Many other cosmetics and skin care companies have followed their example, as reflected in their advertisements proclaiming the virtues of essential oils. But this is nothing new. Fragrant herbs have been used to clear complexions and make hair silky and shiny since before the famous Egyptian beauty Cleopatra had special botanical cosmetics created for her. Certain essential oils stimulate oil production in dry skin and hair. Others slow down overactive oil glands. Many oils also soothe irritated skin.

Why Don't I Like a Scent That Others Enjoy?

Not everyone likes the same fragrances. I know people who feel uncomfortable around cologne or perfume when it is the same one worn by someone they dislike. One man in my class hated the smell of lavender because the funeral parlor in his hometown used it. He came to associate lavender with grief. No matter how many books say that lavender—or any other scent—is relaxing, if you associate its fragrance with bad memories, you may never learn to enjoy it. If so, do not despair: essential oils offer a large selection of appealing fragrances, so you can afford to let one go.

CREATING
FORMULAS:
GETTING STARTED

Making and using essential oil products for healing or skin care is not difficult. Some basic information and a few safety tips are all you need. As you become more familiar with the fragrances and properties of different oils, the process becomes easier. Follow my suggestions in the next five chapters and refer to the descriptions of individual essential oils in the Materia Medica section on page 108. Use your nose as your guide, and do not be afraid to experiment. Take careful notes, and label everything so that you can duplicate effective combinations—or avoid repeating ones that did not work!

Safety

Essential oils are excellent for mind/body health but only when used properly. They are very concentrated. Just one drop of essential oil is roughly equivalent to several cups of herb tea. This estimate varies with each oil, but you can see why it's easy to overdose with essential oil.

- When using essential oils over several months, vary the ones you use to avoid overexposure to any one oil.

- Try to limit your use of essential oils to a few drops a day. That includes the oils in all of your daily products, such as toothpaste, mouthwash, and body lotion. Overdoses tax the liver and kidneys. These organs of elimination are responsible for clearing the body of toxins, including an overload of essential oils.

- Rather than ingesting essential oils, drink herb tea or take capsules or tinctures. Essential oils can burn the inside of your mouth. Since they are quickly absorbed into the mouth and throat—and very little gets to the stomach—when taken orally, they probably will not reach the area you are trying to treat anyway.

- Essential oils can burn or irritate skin, so dilute them in a carrier like vegetable oil before use. Hot oils like cinnamon are especially problematic. Keep essential oils away from your eyes. If you experience skin irritation or accidentally get some in your eyes, flush with straight vegetable oil—not water, which will not dilute essential oils.

- Get fresh air and have adequate ventilation as you work with essential oils to avoid symptoms from overexposure to them. An overdose caused by skin absorption or by smelling them can result in nausea, headache, skin irritation, emotional unease, or a "spaced out" feeling. Use an air filter if necessary when preparing essential oil products and giving an aromatherapy massage.

- If you accidentally spill essential oil on yourself, immediately wipe it off with any type of alcohol to remove the residue. It is a good idea to have herbs that are beneficial to the liver and kidneys, such as burdock, milk thistle, turmeric, and dandelion, on hand in the event of a spill.

- Use essential oils cautiously with anyone who is elderly or convalescing and carefully—or not at all—with people who have liver or kidney problems since they can increase the workload of these organs. Insufficient clearing of essential oils acts like an overdose. Oils that overactivate the nervous system or are potential neurotoxins should not be used with people who have chronic nervous system conditions.

- A few people have allergies or sensitivities to essential oils. If there is any chance of this, run a patch test by mixing one drop of the suspect essential oil in one-quarter teaspoon of vegetable oil. Place a drop in the crook of the arm and wait twelve hours to see if a reaction occurs. Someone who has a known allergy to a certain plant may or may not be allergic to the essential oil from that plant, but it is still better to avoid its use. The same is true for carrier oils in aromatherapy products. When a person is allergic to almonds or coconut, do not use that oil on them.

- Photosensitizing oils react on the skin of some individuals to produce an uneven skin pigmentation. Use these oils carefully—and never in a suntan lotion or facial cream. The most notorious is bergamot, which contains bergaptene, a powerful photosensitizer. Other citrus can be photosensitizing to various degrees.

- Toxic oils are unsuitable for general use. Use semitoxic oils cautiously. Do not use oils from either category for the elderly, children, or pregnant women.

Potential Skin Irritants

Bay rum   *Clove*
Birch   *Oregano*
Cinnamon   *Thyme (except linalol type)*
Citronella

Potential Photosensitizing Essential Oils

Bergamot   *Orange*

Slightly Photosensitizing Essential Oils

Cumin   *Lemon*   *Lime*

Essential Oils to Avoid Because They Are Toxic to the Nervous System (not used in this book)

Calamus
(Acorus calamus)

Camphor
(Cinnamomum camphora)

Mugwort
(Artemesia vulgaris)

Nutmeg
(Myristica fragrans)

Pennyroyal
(Mentha pelugium)

Sassafras
(Sassafras albidum)

Savory
(Satureja hortensis)

Tansy
(Tanacetum annuum)

Thuja
(Thuja occidentalis)

Wormwood
(Artemisia arborescens)

Potentially Semitoxic Essential Oils

Bitter almond
(Prunus amygdalus)

Birch
(Betula lenta)

Hyssop *(Hyssopus officinalis)*

Sage *(Salvia spp.)*

Wintergreen
(Gaultheria hookeri)

Essential Oils to Avoid If You Have Epilepsy

Cajeput
(*Melaluca leucadendra*)

Camphor
(*Cinnamomum camphora*)

Eucalyptus
(*Eucalyptus globulus*)

Fennel
(*Foeniculum vulgare*)

Hyssop
(*Hyssopus officinalis*)

Rosemary
(*Rosmarinus officinalis*)

Sage
(*Salvia spp.*)

Thuja
(*Thuja occidentalis*)

Wormwood
(*Artemisia arborescens*)

Equipment and Supplies

Your kitchen contains almost everything you need to make aromatherapy preparations at home. Measuring cups and spoons, bowls, and pans double as your laboratory equipment. Nut and vegetable oils, such as almond, apricot, grape seed, and coconut, and jojoba wax, as well as essential oils, are available in most natural-food stores, herb shops, and online.

Glass droppers that measure essential oils to transfer into your products are sold in drugstores and some natural-food stores. A dropper is usually accurate enough, although the size of a drop varies slightly depending on the size of the dropper opening, the temperature, and the thickness (viscosity) of the essential oil. It is important not to contaminate essential oils when you move the dropper from one vial of oil to another. Rather than having a separate dropper for each oil, you can rinse the dropper in a small amount of alcohol (such as vodka). Wait a few minutes for the alcohol to completely evaporate before using the dropper again.

Carrier Oils

To make a simple aromatherapy product, add ten to twelve drops of essential oil to an ounce of a carrier, such as almond oil. This is a 2 percent dilution that is suitable for spot therapy in which the finished product is applied to only one area of the body. Half that amount of essential oil (a 1 percent solution) is better for children, pregnant women, and anyone in weak health. The resulting oil can also be used as body, massage, or bath oil. See the Essential Oil Products Dilutions Chart, page 39, for the number of drops you need for different aromatherapy preparations.

Vegetable oils used as carrier oils are heavier and thicker than essential oils. They are absorbed into the skin's top layers, but generally do not penetrate the skin, despite many product claims to the contrary. Unlike essential oils, their molecules are too large to get through. There is some absorption of the vitamin E found in cold-pressed oils. Castor oil seems to be an exception with some of its compounds absorbed, especially when it is thinned with another oil or water.

Specialty carrier oils—such as rose hip oil—containing the fatty acid GLA (gamma linolenic acid) are expensive but maintain healthy skin, repair damage, and reduce inflammation. GLA helps heal psoriasis and eczema, counter allergies, and diminish new wrinkles, stretch marks, and scars. It also relieves stiff joints and may promote the immune system, but only when taken internally.

I generally prefer using unprocessed carrier oils. However, sometimes the strong smell of cold-pressed virgin olive or sesame oil overpowers the aroma of a product, so a lighter oil that has been processed is needed for an aromatherapy effect. Some carrier oils are purposely altered in the laboratory to make them easier to work with and improve the texture of the finished product. Fractionated coconut oil is made by using heat to separate out the long-chain fatty acids and lauric acid. These compounds have high melting points, so they solidify quickly and can be removed when cooled. What remains in the oil are medium-chain fatty caprylic and capric acids that are also antimicrobial. Fractionation results in a tasteless, odorless, and more expensive oil for use in body care products that require a liquid oil that will not harden at room temperatures like unprocessed coconut oil, which is about half lauric acid that has antibacterial, anti-fungal, and antiviral properties.

Popular Carrier Oils

Almond	Coconut	Olive
Apricot	Grape seed	Sesame
Avocado	Hazelnut	
Castor	Jojoba wax	

Specialty Carrier Oils

Black cumin seed	Hazelnut	Rose hip seed
Borage seed	Raspberry seed	Sea buckthorn seed and berry

Incorporating Herbs into Aromatherapy

Combining herbs and essential oils increases their capacity for healing. You can prepare salves, lotions, and creams with essential oils. *Infused oils*, which are made by soaking herbs in vegetable oil, may replace plain vegetable carrier oil to make the medicine more potent. Some examples of popular infused oils are arnica, calendula, and St. John's wort oils, which all heal injured skin. You can purchase infused oils or make your own following the instructions below.

Homemade Infused Carrier Oil

To prepare your own infused carrier oil, place finely chopped fresh or dried herbs in a wide-mouth glass jar, and add just enough of your choice of vegetable oil to completely cover the herbs. (If you use fresh herbs, it's very important to use a very clean jar and have the herb material completely covered to avoid mold.) Stir to remove any air bubbles. Put the jar in a warm place—in a sunny window, a slow cooker set to very low heat (so it does not crack the jar), by a heater, or outdoors in the summer—for one to two days with constant heat or for about four days if the temperature fluctuates. When fully infused, the oil will take on the color and scent of the herbs. Strain the oil through a strainer or cheesecloth, pour into a bottle, and store in a cool place.

Preserving Your Creations

Fortunately, the essential oils themselves serve as excellent preservatives for your homemade aromatherapy products. They are all antibacterial and antifungal to some degree, and most are antioxidants. Some of the strongest natural preservatives are rosemary, tea tree, eucalyptus, and lavender. Adding additional antioxidant vitamins E and/or C further extends the life of essential and vegetable oils. Using very clean equipment and containers will also help. The problem is mostly with creams and lotions since they contain water and are easily contaminated when fingers dip into them. Refrigeration and removing the product with a clean stick or spatula can help. Commercial products rely on synthetic or semisynthetic preservatives to extend their shelf life, whether their labels admit it or not.

Tips for Creating Custom Formulas

The many choices that go into the creation of a blend may seem intimidating, but this adds to the creativity. Every drop you add takes your blend in a direction that is new and interesting. Keep records of ingredients, proportions, processing procedures, and comments. Label your finished products with the ingredients, date, and any special instructions. It is easiest for beginners to use no more than three essential oils in a blend. Do not worry—you can design an effective remedy with just a few oils.

To create an essential oil product, I first decide what physical and emotional properties I want to treat and make a list of the best oils recommended for those conditions. (Refer to descriptions of each oil's use in this book's Materia Medica section, page 108). Then, I work out a formula. You can start out using equal parts of each oil. As your confidence increases, you will find yourself adjusting the proportions and adding a larger percentage of the formula's most important oils. I then turn my attention to making it smell fantastic by readjusting the proportions. At this point, I may decide to use less of an overpowering essential oil or even replace it in favor of a softer one with similar properties to make the final product smell better. Finally, I measure my drops and add them to a carrier. I sniff the new creation along the way to make sure the scent is good. The blend will "mature" and improve over the next few days and weeks. It is good to formulate small amounts in case you need to alter the final product. Be sure to take careful notes of all ingredients so you can do so.

While you're blending, your nose quickly becomes accustomed to the scent so you no longer perceive the blend accurately. Walk away for at least fifteen minutes, then return with a fresh nose. If you have the luxury of creating your blend over several days, take it slow, giving yourself time to make subtle adjustments.

With experience, you'll be able to imagine how the blend will smell while you are designing the formula. Eventually you will even predict the direction the fragrance will take as the individual oils blend together over the next few weeks. Practice is your best instructor when learning how to make essential oil blends. Why do I care that my products smell wonderful? It encourages the enjoyment and more frequent use of the product. I also believe a wonderful scent reaches deeper levels into the psyche for improved healing.

Borrow a few hints from professional perfumers, who consider the *top notes*, *middle notes*, and *low notes*. These terms define how heavy or light the scent appears. A fragrance that is light and airy, like rose or lavender, contains many top notes. Those that are heavy and lingering—patchouli and vetiver, for example—consist of predominantly low notes. The middle notes, found in an herb like marjoram, lie in between. Perfume smells most intriguing when it contains all three notes. While trying to categorize an oil, keep in mind it can contain more than one note.

Essential oils vary in odor intensity, so avoid using too many strongly aromatic essential oils in the same formula until you have enough blending experience to keep them from becoming overpowering. You'll recognize oils with a high odor intensity—such as chamomile, patchouli, cinnamon, ylang-ylang, and clary sage—just by smelling them. Usually, one drop for every ounce of an intense oil like these is sufficient. Go easy on pungent or sharp essential oils.

Combining eucalyptus, tea tree, and rosemary usually smells too sharp and medicinal.

A shortcut for beginning aromatherapists is to start with an essential oil that has a fairly complex chemistry so it already smells like a blend. A good example is geranium, which contains hints of rose, cedarwood, herb, and citrus. To teach your nose about blending, try changing the scent by adding a small amount of another oil with a rose, woodsy, herbal, or citrus scent one drop at a time. Each oil moves the scent into a different direction.

Another blending technique is to choose essential oils that smell similar to each other. This performs a delightful trick on the nose because the oils play off one another, making your blend seem more complicated and mysterious. Try combining small amounts of mints such as peppermint and spearmint, citrus such as lemon and bergamot, or spice scents like cinnamon and ginger.

Regarding Quality

To make a quality product, start with quality essential oils. This is based on purity, growing conditions, differences among species, extraction techniques, and proper storage. The best advice for judging quality is to train your nose. Your sense of smell will become keener as you work with good essential oils. If you can, attend a hands-on aromatherapy seminar. I always warn my students that just one seminar will make their sense of smell so discerning, it spoils them for life because products on the market containing synthetic essential oils will not smell as good as they once did. Budding aromatherapists often realize that some candles, body care products, and air fresheners they already have in their homes are scented with essential oils that have been concocted in a laboratory. Shopping in craft stores and gift shops that smell strongly of synthetic scents from products they carry can become difficult.

Another way to educate your nose is to sniff through a selection of essential oils in a store in order to smell the differences. Do not be shy about asking questions; although some store clerks assume that any product marked "essential oil" is a natural oil made from a plant, there are synthetic essential oils. Some companies who sell essential oils make inaccurate claims and stretch the truth to encourage sales. Many of the most reliable essential oil companies are run by aromatherapists who stake their reputations on supplying good essential oils.

I have worked in the essential oil industry for decades and have seen a lot of marketing techniques. Essential oil companies often use terminology to describe the quality of their oils. Keep in mind that terms such as *high quality*, *therapeutic*, *medicinal grade*, *superior*, and *pure standard* are not standardized terms that are used in the industry. These terms are relevant only to the company using them and do not accurately refer to grades of oils.

Purity

Purity is of concern when purchasing essential oils. Rare and expensive oils are the most likely candidates for adulteration. This can be done by diluting or "extending" them with vegetable oil, alcohol, or another solvent. An essential oil cut with another oil will have different properties. Lemon verbena and melissa (lemon balm) may be mixed with the much cheaper lemongrass, citronella, or lemon eucalyptus. Having an educated and discerning nose will help you sniff out the imposters.

Diluted oils may smell weak and be less expensive. You can determine whether an essential oil has been diluted with vegetable oil by placing a small drop on a piece of paper. Because they evaporate so easily, most essential oils leave no stain, except for the thick oils, such as patchouli, benzoin, German chamomile, and sandalwood. Oils extended by adding alcohol have a slight "boozy" odor. It is more difficult to tell when an essential oil is diluted with an odorless solvent, and this is problematic because solvents can be toxic and are absorbed through the skin and inhaled through the lungs. Your best bet is to purchase your essential oils from a reliable source.

Essential Oil Grades

Many essential oils are available in different grades that reflect their quality. As long as it is pure and natural, you may not always need the highest grade of essential oil for every project. High-grade essential oils carry more of a bouquet, a fuller-bodied fragrance that you learn to detect by working with the oils. When an essential oil like rose or lavender smells different from another one, it does not necessarily mean that one is inferior. Personal preference can be your guide. Low-grade oils can cost more in the long run. A friend who makes facial creams had to use four times as much essential oil to achieve the same fragrance after she switched to an inferior grade.

Avoid Synthetic Oils

Once they smell high-quality essential oils, my aromatherapy students begin to easily sniff out synthetics. Usually made with petroleum-based chemicals, synthetic essential oils attempt to duplicate natural scents, but they rarely come close. They can actually be harmful since their tiny molecules penetrate the skin and enter the bloodstream. When people say that they react adversely or are allergic to a fragrance, I first suspect that they have encountered only synthetics.

Sad to say, synthetic fragrances permeate our lives. Many body-care products—even those sold in natural-food stores—contain them. Most fruits and flowers do not naturally produce essential oils, so when you see "essential oil" of carnation, lily of the valley, strawberry, or gardenia, you can be sure these are synthetics. When choosing skin-care products, read the labels carefully to make sure the essential oils in them have been derived from plants rather than made in a laboratory. One way to tell is to look for the botanical name of each plant listed on the label.

Proper Storage

Once you've gone to the trouble of locating and purchasing quality essential oils, you will want to keep them that way. Store them in dark glass vials with tight lids in a cool place out of direct sunlight. Properly stored, most essential oils will keep for years. Citrus oils, such as orange and lemon, are the most vulnerable to oxidation and spoilage, but even they can last a couple of years if kept in a cool place. A few essential oils—such as patchouli, clary sage, benzoin, vetiver, and sandalwood—actually improve with age. I have forty-year-old patchouli that smells so rich and vanilla-like, people have trouble identifying the fragrance—even those who hate the smell of patchouli often say that they love it. They find it difficult to believe the oil is really patchouli.

I prefer to keep all aromatherapy products in glass containers, but especially pure essential oils, which eventually eat away plastic, contaminating the oil. Plastic inserts or "reducers" that are inserted into the top of the essential oil bottle to release only a drop of essential oil at a time can also be a problem when oils are stored over time.

Supply Checklist

Essential oils (suggestions on page 38)
Carrier (vegetable oils, glycerin, distilled water, or grain alcohol)
Pyrex measuring cup
Clean, empty glass bottles with lids
Measuring spoons
Glass droppers
Small funnel
Notebook, pencil
Labels for bottles

Clean-up supplies

Paper towels
Alcohol

Essential Oil Starter Kit

Oil	For relief of
German Chamomile	indigestion, stress, allergies, rashes, muscle cramps, inflammation, anxiety, anger, and depression
Geranium	imbalance of mind and body
Lavender	infection, inflammation, insomnia, pain, depression, and anxiety
Lemon (or other citrus)	infection, depression, and anxiety
Peppermint	indigestion, sinus congestion, itching, panic, and fatigue
Rosemary	pain, congestion, grief, poor circulation, and forgetfulness
Tea tree or Eucalyptus	infection and fatigue

When I pick or crush in my hand a twig of bay, or brush against a bush of rosemary, or tread upon a tuft of thyme, or pass through incense-laden cistus, I feel that here is all that is best and purest and most refined, and nearest to poetry in the range of faculty of the sense of smell.

—GERTRUDE JEKYLL,
British Garden Designer, 1843–1932

Essential Oil Products Dilutions Chart

Bath oil	10 drops essential oil in 1 ounce carrier oil. Use 1 teaspoon per bath. Or 2–3 drops pure essential oil per bath.
Bath salt	10–12 drops essential oil in ½ cup table or rock salt. Use 1–2 tablespoons per bath.
Body oil	10–12 drops essential oil in 1 ounce carrier oil
Liniment	10–12 drops essential oil in ½ ounce carrier oil. Apply only on sore areas.
Massage oil	6–8 drops essential oil in 1 ounce carrier oil
Perfume	10 drops essential oil in 1 teaspoon brandy. Dab on a few drops.
Potpourri	10–15 drops essential oils in 1 cup dried herbs
Room/facial/body spray	10–12 drops essential oil in 2 ounces water. Shake before using.
Salve/cream/lotion	Stir 10–12 drops into 1 ounce salve or body lotion, or a commercial cream (stirring may break emulsion of homemade cream and separate out water)
Sitz bath	3 drops in basin large enough to sit in. Can also be used as hand or foot soak.
Smelling salts	10–12 drops essential oil in 2 tablespoons table or rock salt. Keep in closed container.
Wash: hand/foot	6 drops in small basin of hot or cold water

AROMATHERAPY
AND EMOTIONAL
HEALTH

Researchers are discovering how pleasant smells make people more willing to negotiate, cooperate, and compromise. They can help take the edge off of many emotional conditions, such as depression, insomnia, and even grief. The following essential oil blends can be made into all sorts of aromatherapy concoctions. The Essential Oil Products Dilutions Chart (see page 39) shows you the number of drops to use of the essential oil blend. Create your own massage or bath oils or a body oil to rub on the skin over a problem area, or make your own room or body spray.

Smelling salts may sound old-fashioned, but they are a convenient way to carry a scent around with you. Salt absorbs oils that are added to it and makes the scent last longer. Allow the scents to blend in a lidded glass jar for a day, then store in a sealed vial to keep in your purse or pocket, ready for you to take a sniff as needed. Smelling salts provide a convenient way to carry around a small amount of scent that will not spill or leak like an essential oil. They are an excellent choice for plane travel.

You can also scent a room with these blends. Add three to six drops of just the pure essential oil blend without a carrier to an essential oil diffuser, potpourri cooker, or pan of lightly simmering water. A drop or two of any of these blends can be placed on curtains, furniture, bedding, and other fabrics. (The essential oils themselves stain only silk material and some synthetics.)

There is jewelry designed to hold essential oils and release the fragrance around you. It is often beads made from clay or another absorbent material. Create your own jewelry by adding a few drops of an essential oil blend to a cloth bracelet.

This subtle aromatherapy technique is practical for health care workers who want to have a positive emotional impact on their patients as well as themselves.

Depression

Certain fragrances affect brain waves in a fashion similar to antidepressant drugs. Italian psychologist Dr. Paolo Rovesti successfully lifted many patients out of depression in the 1970s and 1980s with the citrus scents of orange, bergamot, lemon, and lemon verbena. My favorite citrus is the elegantly scented neroli (orange blossom) essential oil. In addition, a happiness response is produced by the scent of cloves. That means any plant with a clove scent buried in it, such as basil, will serve as an antidepressant. Ruhr University researchers in Germany say a new class of GABA modulators may offer "a scientific basis for aromatherapy." GABA is a brain neurotransmitter that is a natural antidepressant produced in the body. It is encouraged by sniffing German chamomile, lemongrass, rose, or jasmine. Marjoram's fragrance appears to promote feelings of contentment and well-being by adjusting the brain's neurotransmitters. An antidepressive massage oil of lavender and marjoram combined with a small amount of the more energizing eucalyptus, rosemary, and peppermint alleviated depression in a study. In discussing melissa (lemon balm), sixteenth-century herbalist John Gerard said that the smell alone "gladdens the heart."

▌Antidepressant Essential Oils

Bergamot	*Lavender*	*Rose*
Cedarwood	*Lemon*	*Rose geranium*
Chamomile	*Lemon verbena*	*Sandalwood*
Citruses	*Marjoram*	*Thyme*
Clary sage	*Melissa (lemon balm)*	*Vetiver*
Cloves	*Neroli*	*Ylang-ylang*
Geranium	*Orange*	
Helichrysum	*Patchouli*	
Jasmine	*Petitgrain*	

Antidepressant Formula

Try this formula whenever you are feeling down or just need a lift. You can sniff it throughout the day. My favorite suggestion for countering depression is with an aromatic bath that washes away the cares of the world. An aromatherapy massage is always lovely, but you can also rub on a massage oil yourself. Try it after a shower. When you need an antidepressant on the go, carry your aromatherapy spray or smelling salts (see Dilutions Chart, page 39) so they are always available. If you are on antidepressant drugs, feel free to use aromatherapy; there is no evidence that it will interfere.

6 drops bergamot

3 drops petitgrain

3 drops rose geranium

1 drop neroli (orange blossom)
or rose (expensive, so optional)

Combine the essential oils and add the mixture to one ounce of vegetable oil or one ounce of water.

Anxiety

Aromatherapists use several fragrances, such as lavender and German chamomile, to help overcome feelings of anxiety, loneliness, and rejection. These same oils are useful when undergoing major life transitions, such as changing a job or when ending a relationship. Most scents that ease depression also help with anxiety. Antianxiety scents have been used successfully to relax patients in a number of medical settings that include dental offices, neurology clinics, and MRI scanning, as well as for stressed-out nurses working in the emergency room. Essential oils have also been put on the masks of patients going under anesthesia. Studies show this aromatic technique reduces panic attacks, epileptic seizures, and nervousness. Sixteenth-century herbalist John Gerard said that sniffing marjoram helped those "given to much sighing."

You can program your mind to relax before going out into settings that cause you anxiety. First, find a calming environment where you can listen to relaxing music and perhaps have a massage while smelling the blend. Whenever you inhale that aroma in the future, you will associate it with relaxation and feel less anxious. Carrying around a small vial of smelling salts (see Dilutions Chart, page 39) means your antianxiety blend is handy whenever you need a sniff.

Essential Oils to Relieve Anxiety

Basil	Geranium	Peppermint
Bergamot	Juniper	Petitgrain
Cardamom	Lavender	Rose
Chamomile	Marjoram	Rosemary
Cypress	Melissa (lemon balm)	Sandalwood
Fennel	Neroli	Vanilla
Frankincense	Orange	

Antianxiety Formula

This blend calms your mind and helps you refocus. A spray is handy to carry so it is available to calm you down at the first uncomfortable signs of nervousness or anxiousness.

6 drops lavender

3 drops orange

1 drop marjoram

1 drop geranium

Combine the essential oils and add the mixture to one ounce of vegetable oil or one ounce of water.

Fatigue

In a study, computer operators made fewer mistakes when inhaling eucalyptus or peppermint. The scent of both essential oils was shown to stimulate brain waves. There are alarm clocks that awaken sleepers by dispensing scents that make one feel more alert, such as eucalyptus and pine. Lemon, cypress, and peppermint are circulated through corporate air-conditioning systems throughout the workday to keep employees more attentive—and reduce their urge to smoke. The spicy aromas of clove, basil, black pepper, cinnamon, and to a lesser degree, patchouli, rose, sage, and lemongrass reduce drowsiness, irritability, and headaches. They have been found to prevent the sharp drop in attention typical after thirty minutes of work—without over-amping the adrenal glands as caffeine does. In the early 1920s, Italian doctor-researchers Giovanni Gatti and Renato Cayola found that clove, cinnamon, lemon, cardamom, and fennel made their patients feel more alert and responsive. Basil, jasmine, peppermint, and rosemary appear to stimulate the brain's beta waves that focus mental activity, awareness, and alertness—and make you feel good. They slow breathing by blocking stress-related nerve responses but without depressing the nervous system. Sixteenth-century herbalist John Gerard said that clary sage counters mental fatigue and nervous disorders.

Stimulating Essential Oils

Basil	*Fennel*	*Lemongrass*
Cinnamon	*Jasmine*	*Peppermint*
Clary sage	*Lavender*	*Rosemary*
Eucalyptus	*Lemon*	*Tea tree*

Stimulant Formula

We all encounter times when we need to perk up and be more alert. A few sniffs of this blend should help you wake up. It will help you stay attentive after a short night of sleep or when working on late-night projects. The good news is that it will not interfere with sleep; just discontinue use an hour beforehand. To stay alert while driving, spray it in your car or on a small piece of cardboard to hang from your car's mirror.

> 7 drops lemon
>
> 2 drops eucalyptus
>
> 2 drops peppermint
>
> 1 drop lemongrass

Combine the essential oils and add the mixture to one ounce of vegetable oil or one ounce of water.

Poor Memory

Memory is enhanced with aroma. I keep a sprig of rosemary next to my computer to increase concentration. Research confirms that rosemary's scent is a brain stimulant, as are peppermint and bay laurel. Sage seems to slow short-term memory loss by blocking certain brain pathways that cause poor recall. In one study, volunteers memorized words more easily when they sniffed jasmine. Researchers have learned that mental recall improves dramatically when a past event is associated with a certain aroma. Familiar fragrances can send you back in time, evoking long-forgotten images and feelings. In the 1960s, French psychologist Jean Valnet found vanilla helped his patients unlock childhood memories.

Memory-Stimulating Essential Oils

Bay laurel	*Peppermint*	*Thyme*
Clove bud	*Rosemary*	
Fennel	*Sage*	

Memory Formula

For a memory boost, make body oil or cologne to dab on your temples or elsewhere while studying or working. You'll thank yourself at that test or meeting later! This is the perfect blend to make into smelling salts (see Dilutions Chart, page 39) for sniffing when you are trying to recall that important fact. Lavender is added to the formula below to help increase mental focus and sweeten the overall scent.

5 drops lavender

4 drops bay laurel

3 drops rosemary

1 drop peppermint

Combine the essential oils and add the mixture to one ounce of vegetable oil or one ounce of water.

Grief

In Europe, the scents of sage, clary sage, and rosemary were said to help people overcome grief. Lavender is traditional to comfort the sick or anyone feeling emotionally upset. In the sixteenth century, herbalist John Gerard wrote that basil "taketh away sorrowfulness . . . and maketh a man merry and glad" and suggested a whiff of marjoram "for those given to much sighing" due to grief, loneliness, or rejection. Ancient Egyptians, Greeks, and Romans also sniffed marjoram to gain emotional strength. The Greeks used cypress and hyssop, and several other ancient cultures burned sandalwood at death ceremonies to comfort mourners and appease both the living and departed. Grief and sadness are natural parts of life. Aroma has long been used to help an individual feel better. A traditional way to use grief-resolving formulas was to place the fragrance on a hanky. If overcome with emotion, the individual could politely bring the scented hanky up to the face and inhale deeply. You can revive the hanky tradition by lightly scenting facial tissues. Place 10 drops of the essential oil blend on the top of a cardboard box of tissues. Enclose the box in a sealed plastic bag and leave it for about three days to allow the scent to disperse, then remove it. If that is too much work, simply make smelling salts or bath oil.

Essential Oils to Ease Grief

Cypress	*Juniper*	*Rose*
Frankincense	*Marjoram*	*Rosemary*

Grief-Resolving Formula

Geranium is not considered specifically for grief, but it has a very balancing effect on emotions and softens and pulls this formula together.

> 6 drops geranium
>
> 3 drops rose
>
> 1 drop marjoram
>
> 1 drop cypress or rosemary

Combine the essential oils and add the mixture to one ounce of vegetable oil or one ounce of water.

Insomnia

Lack of sleep is a problem for millions of Americans, often leading to tiredness, poor concentration, agitation, depression, dizziness, and headaches. Clinical studies show that people get a better night's sleep with good smells and wake up feeling more invigorated and satisfied. Lavender's aroma increases deep, slow-wave sleep with less restlessness. In some studies, it worked as well as pharmaceutical sleeping pills. Aromas that enhance the brain neurotransmitter GABA encourage relaxation and sleep, sometimes even more than sleeping pills do. Rose, German chamomile, and lemongrass go right to the brain to lull you to sleep. If you get caught in the repetitive cycle called "looping" and anxious thoughts prevent you from sleep, also try the essential oils suggested under Anxiety (see page 45).

Essential Oils for Insomnia

Chamomile	*Neroli (orange blossom)*
Frankincense	*Petitgrain*
Jasmine	*Rose*
Lavender	*Sandalwood*
Lemon verbena	*Ylang-ylang*
Marjoram	
Melissa (lemon balm)	

Sleep Formula

An excellent way to encourage sleep is a relaxing bath oil of this blend used right before bed. Another good use of this blend is to fill a small pillow with sleep-promoting herbs as a potpourri. (Sew two squares of fabric together on three sides to make a pouch, then fill it with herbs and add a few drops of the essential oil blend. Sew the fourth side shut and you'll have a homemade aromatherapy sleep pillow.) Or, a quicker method is to dab the essential oil blend on the fabric of a small pillow. Seal the pillow in a zip-top plastic bag for a few days so the scent can permeate it, then keep it on your bed, ready to grab and sniff whenever insomnia strikes. I always travel with my four- by six-inch aromatherapy pillow as part of my sleep kit.

> 6 drops bergamot
>
> 1 drop German chamomile
>
> 3 drops geranium
>
> 1 drop frankincense
>
> 1 drop rose

Combine the essential oils and add the mixture to one ounce of vegetable oil or one ounce of water.

Stress and Nervousness

Fragrance can lower rapid pulse and breathing. Researchers from the International Flavors and Fragrances corporation even patented a blend of neroli, valerian, and nutmeg to ease workplace stress. In a study, people in a room scented with lavender, bergamot, marjoram, sandalwood, lemon, or

German chamomile tended to mingle more and be less competitive with each other. Their brain-wave reaction indicated that the scent produced a relaxing effect. Studies show that these same scents enhance relaxation, promote sleep, and help to relieve depression. Twentieth-century Italian researchers Giovanni Gatti and Renato Cayola found that the most sedating oils were neroli, petitgrain, chamomile, valerian, and a low-grade myrrh called opopanax. Sniffing valerian, along with the related spikenard, increases the calming and meditative theta brain waves and deeply relaxing delta waves while decreasing the more stimulating beta waves. Neroli, lavender, and rosemary aromas have been shown to lower cortisol levels brought up by stress. "Green odors" such as these also help protect the body from negative effects of stress. The combination of peppermint, helichrysum, and basil proved especially useful in one study to overcome stress burnout. In another study, massage oil that included marjoram and ylang-ylang dropped both cortisol and blood pressure levels.

Essential Oils to Reduce Stress

Basil	*Frankincense*	*Neroli*
Bergamot	*Helichrysum*	*Orange*
Cardamom	*Jasmine*	*Petitgrain*
Cedarwood	*Juniper*	*Rose*
Chamomile	*Lavender*	*Sandalwood*
Cinnamon	*Lemon*	*Valerian*
Clary sage	*Lemon verbena*	*Vanilla*
Clove	*Marjoram*	*Ylang-ylang*
Eucalyptus	*Melissa (lemon balm)*	
Fennel	*Myrrh*	

Sedative Formula

Sniff this formula at the office, at home when the kids are bouncing off the walls, or whenever life seems overwhelming. It will help reduce emotional stress. Using this sedative blend as a massage oil offers the ultimate aromatherapy relaxation experience. The next best is as bath oil. I also like this formula as an aromatherapy spray for work, in the car, and at home, or as an air freshener—even spray it directly on yourself. Just be sure to close your eyes!

4 drops lavender

2 drops sandalwood or cedarwood

2 drops bergamot

1 drop German chamomile

1 drop ylang-ylang

2 drops petitgrain

Combine the essential oils and add the mixture to one ounce of vegetable oil or one ounce of water.

Sedative Formula for Kids

5 drops lavender

2 drops bergamot

2 drops German chamomile

3 drops lemon or grapefruit

Combine the essential oils and add the mixture to one ounce of vegetable oil or one ounce of water.

Aphrodisiacs

Research tells us that many of the fragrances known traditionally as aphrodisiacs both stimulate and relax brain waves. Need to relax your partner? Ylang-ylang, rose, patchouli, sandalwood, and jasmine relieve stress but are still considered stimulating aphrodisiacs. Men favor lavender and food-related scents like cinnamon, but that essential oil can burn, so it's not suggested for an erotic massage oil. Use it in a room spray or an essential oil diffuser instead. Women tend to be more turned on by floral scents and vanilla.

Aphrodisiac Essential Oils

Black pepper	*Ginger*	*Rose*
Cardamom	*Jasmine*	*Vanilla*
Cinnamon	*Patchouli*	*Ylang-ylang*

Aphrodisiac Formula

Want a little spark in your love life? The first aromatherapy product that comes to mind is massage oil, although this blend should do the trick no matter how it is used.

8 drops jasmine

8 drops vanilla

2 drops ylang-ylang

1 drop cardamom

Combine the essential oils and add the mixture to one ounce of vegetable oil or one ounce of water.

Spiritual Connection

Ancient cultures worldwide have regarded incense as a mediator between worshipper and deity. Strong aromas with "heavenly" scents were used to aid purification. Prayers were sent into the smoke from the burning incense to communicate between the worlds. A special reverence was given to trees, for they seemed to join earth and sky, representing the mundane with the divine. Rosemary and marjoram represented both birth and death, so they were included in both weddings and funerals. Lavender is still burned with heavier resins such as myrrh in some Greek Orthodox churches. Sandalwood, frankincense, myrrh, cedarwood (including the famous cedars of Lebanon), juniper, cypress, and camphor are trees considered sacred by ancient cultures.

Essential Oils to Enhance Spirituality

Cedarwood	*Lavender*	*Rosemary*
Cypress	*Marjoram*	*Sandalwood*
Frankincense	*Myrrh*	
Juniper	*Rose*	

Spiritual Anointing Formula

4 drops sandalwood

2 drops cedarwood

3 drops lavender

1 drop frankincense

1 drop myrrh

Combine the essential oils and add the mixture to one ounce of vegetable oil or one ounce of water.

AROMATHERAPY
SKIN CARE AND
HAIR CARE

Choose techniques and essential oils for your skin care based on your complexion type. The main types are (1) mature complexion that is generally dry, (2) oily skin, (3) "problem" complexion, associated with blackheads and acne, and (4) normal complexion. When your complexion falls into more than one category, treat this "combination" complexion with several techniques. Keep in mind that essential oils will not only improve your complexion, but their aroma will also help to balance your emotions.

Facial Techniques

A facial is one of the kindest things you can give your complexion. The complete treatment includes cleansing, steaming, and exfoliating with a mask, topped off with a facial toner or cream. All of these techniques increase circulation, giving your face a healthful and radiant glow. The entire facial, but especially the skin toners, may also be used for an all-over body treatment.

Cleansing

Remove any makeup with a water-soluble cleansing cream that does not strip off natural skin oils. Then, thoroughly cleanse your face. Soap can be harsh because it makes your skin temporarily alkaline. Ground oats mixed with enough water to create a creamy consistency is a good cleansing alternative. Add a drop of your choice of essential oil that is appropriate for your complexion type to the oatmeal "cream," and gently scrub your face with it, then rinse. If an oily complexion requires more scrubbing, add a little cornmeal to the oatmeal. Do not scrub too much, or your skin will be encouraged to produce more oil, and it will aggravate acne. Avoid products containing abrasive almond husk. Cleanse oily or problem skin twice daily, dry skin only once a day.

Facial Scrub

This scrub will revitalize your skin, leaving you feeling ready to face the day—or night. You can keep a small amount next to your sink and use it on your face instead of soap.

>   3 tablespoons oats
>
>   1 tablespoon cornmeal (optional)
>
>   Water, tea, or hydrosol to moisten

Grind the oats and cornmeal (if using) in an electric coffee grinder. Store the powder in a closed container. To use the scrub, moisten 1 teaspoon with enough water, tea, or hydrosol to make a paste. Apply to your dampened face. Gently scrub and rinse with warm water.

Steaming

Steaming is a mini sauna for your face. Besides cleansing and leaving your face looking youthful and vibrant, it moisturizes skin and unclogs pores. The heat increases circulation and cell metabolism. Steaming may be done a few times a week unless your complexion is extremely dry or delicate. If so, restrict steaming to five minutes every other week. Avoid steaming altogether if you have couperose skin that easily reddens from small, broken blood vessels just under the skin's surface.

Facial Steam

This facial steam will give both your skin and your mood a much-needed lift.

> 1 quart water
>
> 3 drops lavender
>
> 3 drops rosemary
>
> 3 drops geranium

As soon as you bring the water to a simmer in a saucepan, remove it from the heat, and add the essential oils. Holding your face about 12 inches above the pan, place a bath towel over the back of your head, and tuck the ends around the pan to enclose your face in a miniature sauna. Be sure to keep your eyes closed so they will not be irritated by the essential oils. Steam for a few minutes, then remove your head and take a few breaths of fresh air. Go back under the towel and repeat a few times. (Steam for no longer than 5 to 10 minutes per session—less if you have sensitive skin.)

The Facial Mask

A facial mask is a type of gentle exfoliation that is better for skin than the chemical exfoliants used in beauty salons. The mask removes dead skin cells from the skin's surface, uncovering young, fresh skin, and stimulates growth of underlying cells. It also draws water from underlying levels to the skin's surface. This temporarily plumps up skin, magically reducing enlarged pores and wrinkles. Astringent, clay masks are suitable for oily or normal skin conditions.

An oatmeal or cream of wheat mask is less drawing. Gentler masks with honey, avocado, egg whites, and/or fresh fruits such as papaya and yogurt are preferred for a delicate or dry complexion. You can add finely ground, skin-healing herbs, such as rosemary, or rose petals, to any mask. The herbs can be ground in a spice or coffee grinder.

Exfoliating Mask

Your face will thank you if you can take the time to use this natural mask once a week.

> 1 tablespoon finely ground oats or clay powder
>
> 1 teaspoon honey, slightly heated
>
> 1 to 2 teaspoons aloe vera juice or an herb tea
>
> 1 drop lavender

Mash the oats or clay with the honey and aloe to form a thin paste. Stir in the lavender. Apply to your face in an even layer, avoiding sensitive areas around your eyes and mouth. Leave on for 5 to 30 minutes, or as long as is comfortable. (Do not allow the mask to dry or pull so much that it becomes irritating.) Finally, wash the mask off with warm water and gently pat your face dry.

Complexion Toner

Toners are suitable for both dry and oily complexions. Astringent toners offer oily and problem skins a good alternative to oil-based moisturizers, and they double as a men's aftershave. Using aloe vera or a hydrosol in a toner moisturizes the skin and helps heal damaged cells. Vinegar balances the skin's pH and is a natural, protective mantle that relieves itching and flakiness. I like apple cider vinegar because it contains more minerals than refined vinegar, but any vinegar will work. Alcohol and commercial witch hazel (which contains alcohol) are too drying for all but the oiliest complexions. Even then, use only a small amount since alcohol can cause the skin to compensate by producing even more oil.

Cream or Lotion

Creams are ideal for dry or mature complexions. They contain water, so they moisturize skin and protect it from the environment. For oily skin, use a toner or a light lotion instead of a cream. Just a little oil encourages skin to cut down on its own oil production.

Skin Care by Complexion Type

Essential Oils for All Skin Types

Chamomile	*Jasmine*	*Rose*
Clary sage	*Lavender*	*Rosemary*
Geranium	*Palmarosa*	

Dry Skin

A number of essential oils balance skin-oil production, reduce puffiness, and rejuvenate skin by encouraging new cell growth. The classic antiaging ingredients are lavender, geranium, neroli (orange blossom), rosemary, and rose. Peppermint is usually considered drying to skin, but a small amount—say a drop in a formula—actually encourages oil production.

Essential Oils for Dry Skin

Carrot seed	*Lavender*	*Rosemary*
Chamomile	*Neroli*	*Sandalwood*
Clary sage	*Palma rosa*	*Vetiver*
Frankincense	*Patchouli*	*Ylang-ylang*
Geranium	*Peppermint*	
Jasmine	*Rose*	

Oily Skin

For oily skin, use essential oils that normalize overactive sebaceous glands, slowing oil production.

Essential Oils for Oily Skin

Basil	*Eucalyptus*	*Palma rosa*
Bergamot	*Geranium*	*Rose*
Cedarwood	*Juniper*	*Tea tree*
Chamomile	*Lavender*	*Ylang-ylang*
Clary sage	*Lemongrass*	
Cypress	*Lemon verbena*	

The world is a rose; smell it and pass it to your friend.

PERSIAN PROVERB

Toner for Oily Skin

Without the ylang-ylang, which is too sweet-smelling for most men (and some women!), this makes an excellent aftershave for men.

    5 drops cedarwood

    3 drops lemon

    1 drop ylang-ylang

    1 tablespoon aloe vera

    2 ounces witch hazel

Combine the ingredients in a jar with a lid. Shake well before using. Apply with cotton pads.

Cleanser for Oily Skin

If it's available, you can use an herbal vinegar, such as yarrow, basil, or sage.

    1 teaspoon vinegar

    1 teaspoon glycerin

    6 drops lemon

    2 drops cypress

    2 ounces witch hazel

Blend the ingredients in a jar with a lid. Shake well before each use. Apply with cotton pads, then rinse off.

Problem Skin

Problem skin tends toward acne and can be either oily or dry or even a combination of the two. Many essential oils for problem skin are both antiseptic and drying, so choose ones that are suited for your complexion.

Essential Oils for Problem Skin

Basil	*Helichrysum*	*Patchouli*
Carrot	*Juniper*	*Peppermint*
Chamomile	*Lavender*	*Rosemary*
Clary sage	*Lemon*	*Sage*
Eucalyptus	*Lemongrass*	*Sandalwood*
Frankincense	*Neroli*	*Tea tree*
Geranium	*Palmarosa*	*Thyme*

Blemish Remover

The lavender in this natural acne solution is antiseptic and anti-inflammatory.

1 teaspoon Epsom salt

¼ cup distilled water

4 drops lavender

Place the Epsom salt in a small bowl. Bring the water to a boil and pour it over the salt. When the salt has dissolved, add the lavender. Soak a small absorbent cloth in the solution and press this compress onto the pimple. In a minute or two, as it starts to cool, place the cloth back in the hot water, then reapply. Repeat several times.

Intensive Treatment for Acne

This formula is for those trouble spots you need to take care of—fast!

> 10 drops tea tree
>
> ½ teaspoon powdered clay goldenseal root
>
> Distilled water

Combine the tea tree and goldenseal root in a small bowl. Add distilled water to create a paste. This formula is very concentrated, so apply it directly only on acne spots no more than three times a day. Let it dry and remain on the skin for at least 20 minutes. Rinse.

Hair Care

Whether you have dry, normal, or oily hair, essential oils have something to offer. In addition to making shampoos and hair rinse, you can brush two drops of essential oil directly through your hair. It is therapeutic, but it is also true that hair holds fragrance even better than skin does, making you fragrant for hours.

Essential Oils for All Hair Types

Cedarwood	*Geranium*	*Rose*
Chamomile	*Lavender*	*Rosemary*
Clary sage	*Patchouli*	

▍Essential Oils for Dry Hair

Peppermint   *Sandalwood*

Rosewood   *Ylang-ylang*

▍Essential Oils for Oily Hair

Basil   *Lemon*   *Tea tree*

Cypress   *Lemongrass*

Juniper   *Sage*

▍Essential Oils for Dandruff

Geranium   *Patchouli*   *Tea tree*

Juniper   *Rosemary*   *Ylang-ylang*

Lavender   *Sage*

▍Essential Oils to Slow Hair Loss

Geranium   *Patchouli*   *Ylang-ylang*

Juniper   *Rosemary*

Lavender   *Sage*

Herbal Shampoo

Use a mild and pH-balanced shampoo as the base
for this recipe. Baby shampoos, which generally are
derived from olive and soy oils, are a good choice.

> 2 ounces strong herb tea (your choice)
>
> 2 ounces unscented shampoo
>
> ¼ teaspoon essential oil (your choice)

After straining and cooling the tea, add it to the
shampoo base, then add the essential oil. Shake
well before using.

Herbal Hair Rinse

This rinse is used in place of a hair conditioner. It
balances the pH after shampooing, reversing the
electrical charge so your hair does not have a flyaway
look, and removes shampoo residues, leaving hair
shiny and soft.

> 1 to 2 drops essential oil (your choice)
>
> 1 cup water or herb tea
>
> 2 tablespoons vinegar or lemon juice

Combine all of the ingredients. Shake very well and
pour over your scalp and hair after shampooing.
Leave on for several minutes, then rinse. This amount
provides enough rinse to use one to two times. Lemon
juice is used to lighten blonde hair or more likely
provide highlights. However, it is too diluted in this
recipe to do much.

Bathing

Bathing with essential oils is the ultimate aromatherapy experience for both your skin and emotions.

Floating Aromatic Bath Oil

The essential and vegetable oils in this formula float on the surface of the water and make your bath smell heavenly. They also make the water feel smooth, almost creamy. When you emerge, the oils lightly cling to your skin, scenting you for hours. For babies, use only a few drops of this bath oil in the basin. Because this formula contains vegetable oil, it can leave a ring of residue around the inside of your bathtub that requires a little extra cleaning. I find the bathing experience is worth it, but you can have an aromatic bathing experience (without quite the same sensation) by adding only 2 to 3 drops of the pure essential oils to your bath and eliminating the vegetable oil.

8 to 12 drops essential oil (your choice)

1 ounce vegetable oil

Combine the ingredients. Use 1 to 2 teaspoons per bath.

Aromatic Bath Salts

Bath salts are another luxurious addition to your bathwater, making the water feel silky, removing body oils and perspiration, softening the skin, relaxing the muscles, and soaking away the stresses of the day. For muscular aches and pains, add ½ cup Epsom salt to this recipe. All of the salts mentioned in this book can be found at the grocery store.

    1 cup sea salt

    ½ cup borax

    ½ cup baking soda

    ½ teaspoon essential oil (your choice)

Mix the salt, borax, and baking soda together and add the essential oil, mixing well to combine. Use ¼ to ½ cup of the bath salts per bath.

---

*We can complain because rose bushes have thorns,
or rejoice because thorn bushes have roses.*

—ABRAHAM LINCOLN

HEALING THE
BODY WITH
ESSENTIAL OILS

Most essential oils are germ fighters, but their beneficial properties do not stop there. Many heal the skin, aid digestion, or help to stimulate circulation. It is a good idea to incorporate other forms of complementary healing—herbs, bodywork, diet, and lifestyle changes—into your healing regime along with aromatherapy.

When using aromatherapy to treat physical ailments, stick to simple disorders that you would self-diagnose and treat at home anyway, such as a minor sore throat or a bout of indigestion. Think of the remedies in this section as over-the-counter preparations. For more serious problems, seek the advice of a health professional, preferably one skilled in holistic healing. When treating internal problems, diluted essential oils are usually applied externally, right over the problem area to concentrate them where they are needed. The tiny essential oil molecules go through the skin and into the bloodstream. Massage oil designed to ease a stomachache, for example, is rubbed directly over the abdomen; a vapor oil rub on the chest will penetrate into the lungs.

Hives

Hives—rashlike skin bumps that can drive kids (as well as their parents) crazy with itching—are often a symptom of food allergy. You can stop the itching with essential oils, but you should also address the dietary cause of the problem. Wash the skin with an aromatherapy wash and/or use an herbal poultice.

Hives Skin Wash

If you do not have elderflower or calendula to make
the tea, use plain water. This wash can be applied
warm or cold, depending on what feels better. If
the area looks very red, cold water will reduce the
inflammation.

2½ cups water

¼ cup chopped elderflower
or calendula flowers

3 tablespoons baking soda

8 drops lavender

2 drops German chamomile

Bring the water to a boil and pour it over the elder-
flowers. Steep for 15 minutes, then strain out the solids.
Stir in the baking soda and essential oils. Soak a soft
cloth or skin sponge in the solution while stirring to
keep the oils distributed in the water. Apply the cloth
or sponge to irritated skin. Keep the water in a jar in the
refrigerator. Reapply often until itching is alleviated.

Hives Skin Poultice

You may find that even children who normally object to having a treatment smeared on their skin will not mind this one at all—once they know it stops the itching.

> 3 tablespoons bentonite clay
>
> 1 tablespoon slippery elm bark or marshmallow powder
>
> ¼ cup Hives Skin Wash (see opposite)

In a bowl, combine the clay and herb powder. Add the hive wash and stir to make a paste. Set aside for 20 minutes to thicken. Apply to irritated skin with your fingers or a tongue depressor. Let dry on skin. Leave for at least 30 minutes before washing off or reapplying more poultice over the now dried poultice.

Immune System Activity

A number of essential oils encourage immune system activity, increase the rate of new cell growth and healing, and fight infection. These oils work best when used with herbal remedies that aid the immune system.

One important way to assist your immune system is with an aromatherapy lymphatic massage. This involves deep strokes that move cellular fluid through the system, cleansing the body to remove waste. Lymph nodes in the throat, groin, and breasts, under the arms, and elsewhere are filtering centers for the blood. Some massage specialists feel lymph massage is appropriate for people with cancer, especially while undergoing chemotherapy.

Essential Oils for the Immune System

Bergamot	*Lavender*	*Thyme*
Cinnamon	*Lemon*	
Eucalyptus	*Tea tree*	

Essential Oils to Encourage New Cell Growth

Geranium	*Rose*
Lavender	*Sandalwood*

Immune and Anti-Infection Blend

Use this blend as a general massage oil over areas of the body that tend to develop infection. For example, if you get a lot of chest colds and flu, rub this blend over your chest as a preventive measure or at the first signs of illness.

6 drops lavender

6 drops bergamot

3 drops tea tree

2 ounces vegetable oil

Combine all of the ingredients. Massage over appropriate area.

Essential Oils to Stimulate the Lymph System

Bay laurel	*Lavender*	*Orange*
Grapefruit	*Lemon*	*Rosemary*

Lymph Massage Oil

These are among the best essential oils to address the lymphatic system and use for lymphatic massage.

> 6 drops lemon
>
> 6 drops rosemary
>
> 6 drops grapefruit
>
> 3 drops bay laurel
>
> 2 ounces vegetable oil

Combine all of the ingredients. Massage into the body with deep strokes, especially around an area where there is infection. Consider getting a massage from someone who is skilled in lymphatic massage.

Indigestion

The same essential oils that make food tasty help you digest the meals they flavor. Simply inhaling the aromas of these herbs signals the brain to begin a chain reaction that causes your stomach to start grumbling in anticipation. Digestive fluids are pumped into the digestive tract to help you assimilate food.

A massage oil containing essential oils to aid digestion helps relieve belching, stomach pains, and intestinal gas. German chamomile, fennel, and melissa (lemon balm) relax the stomach and soothe burning irritation and inflammation. Peppermint and ginger ease nausea and motion sickness. To overcome nausea, even due to chemotherapy, try basil. Just sniffing ginger or cardamom can be enough to settle a queasy stomach. Cumin relieves headaches from indigestion, rosemary improves poor food absorption, and lemongrass eases nervous indigestion. Peppermint treats irritable bowel syndrome when taken in enteric capsules, which do not open until they reach the intestine. Besides using essential oils externally, you can also turn to ingesting the herbs themselves by sprinkling pepper on your food, serving a peppermint and chamomile tea, or chewing on a juniper berry before meals.

Digestive Aids

Basil	Lavender	Rose
Chamomile	Lemongrass	Rosemary
Cinnamon	Lemon verbena	Thyme
Fennel	Marjoram	
Ginger	Melissa (lemon balm)	
Juniper	Peppermint	

Digestive Massage Oil

This all-purpose formula will help improve the appetite and digestion while preventing nausea. This is a good treatment for anyone who has trouble swallowing medicine, such as young children. You do not need to know fancy massage techniques; simply rub the oil on the belly.

4 drops ginger

3 drops lemongrass

3 drops peppermint

2 drops fennel

2 ounces vegetable oil

Combine all of the ingredients. Rub onto abdomen.

Children's Bath for Indigestion

This bath is perfect for little ones who tend to get upset tummies. The aroma of German chamomile is relaxing, and the other two oils will help put them in a good mood! Chamomile is an expensive essential oil, so if you prefer, replace the chamomile oil in this formula with ½ cup chamomile tea.

1 drop lemongrass

1 drop grapefruit

1 drop German chamomile

Add the essential oils directly to bathwater. Stir to distribute on the water's surface before your child gets into the tub.

Infections

Almost all essential oils are more or less antiseptic, destroying bacteria, fungi, yeast, parasites, and/or viruses. Use essential oils as preventive medicine in your bath or as a body oil. To make a body oil, add 12 drops of your choice of essential oils to 1 ounce of a carrier oil, such as olive oil. Apply over the infected area. Do not use this on large open wounds.

Antibacterial Essential Oils

Basil	*Helichrysum*	*Orange*
Bay laurel	*Lavender*	*Peppermint*
Bergamot	*Lemon*	*Sage*
Clove	*Lemongrass*	*Tea tree*
Eucalyptus	*Marjoram*	*Thyme*
Geranium	*Myrrh*	

Antibacterial Formula

This formula combines antiseptic power for physical relief with soothing scents for emotional relief—the perfect combination!

8 drops tea tree

3 drops lavender

1 ounce vegetable oil

Combine the essential oils with the vegetable oil. Rub the oil over the infected area a few times per day.

Antifungal Essential Oils

Basil	*Frankincense*	*Peppermint*
Bergamot	*Geranium*	*Tea tree*
Cinnamon	*Lemongrass*	*Thyme*
Clove	*Melissa (lemon balm)*	
Eucalyptus	*Myrrh*	

Antifungal Powder

A drying fungal powder or vinegar provides the best base for treating fungal infections like athlete's foot. Small amounts of peppermint diminish the itching of a fungal infection. If you prefer a liquid formula, add these same ingredients (without the bentonite clay) to ½ cup apple cider vinegar, and dab on the afflicted area.

10 drops tea tree or eucalyptus

6 drops geranium

1 drop peppermint

2 tablespoons bentonite clay powder

Drop the essential oils into the clay and mix well. Apply to the problem area.

Anti-Candida Essential Oils

Bergamot	*Lavender*	*Thyme*
Chamomile	*Spearmint*	
Clove	*Tea tree*	

Anti-Infection Douche

The yogurt in this formula helps support and reestablish the natural flora of the vagina and keeps the essential oils evenly distributed throughout the water. The vinegar keeps the region acidic to help deter infection. Douching puts the essential oils in direct contact with the yeast or bacteria causing the infection. When you douche, be sure that the bag is no higher than your head to keep the pressure from being too strong. You can add 6 drops (total) of these same essential oils (without the yogurt) to a bath or a sitz bath. Of the anti-candida essential oils listed above, lavender and tea tree are the only two recommended for a douche. The other oils on the list are too irritating to sensitive areas.

    3 drops lavender

    3 drops tea tree

    3 cups warm water

    2 heaping tablespoons plain,
    unsweetened yogurt (optional)

    3 cups water

    2 tablespoons vinegar

Combine all of the ingredients in a douche bag. Mix well. Use this douche once a day during an active infection.

Antiviral Essential Oils

Bay laurel	*Geranium*	*Peppermint*
Bergamot	*Juniper*	*Rosemary*
Black pepper	*Lavender*	*Tea tree*
Cinnamon	*Lemon*	*Thyme*
Eucalyptus	*Melissa (lemon balm)*	

Herpes and Shingles Formula

If applied to herpes or shingles as soon as the blisters begin to appear, the essential oils in this formula often prevent the breakout. Resist the temptation to apply them undiluted. In addition to tea tree, myrrh, and geranium, other excellent oils to use are eucalyptus (especially lemon eucalyptus) and lavender. Treat these conditions externally by diluting essential oil in an equal amount of vegetable oil or alcohol. This is highly concentrated, so apply it only on the wart or blister.

10 drops tea tree (especially chemotype MQV)

8 drops myrrh

6 drops geranium

½ ounce vegetable oil

Combine all of the ingredients. Apply to only the affected area about four times per day. This is a concentrated formula, so be sure to apply no more than six times a day.

In addition, research shows that creams containing capsaicin, a compound in cayenne, deaden the pain of herpes and shingles. Purchase these at a drugstore, or add cayenne essential oil to a cream base. Go easy, as too much can burn the skin.

Wart Oil

Warts are caused by a viral infection. Castor oil alone can be used on warts, but it is even better to combine it with an antiviral essential oil, such as tea tree.

> 12 drops tea tree
>
> ¼ ounce castor oil
>
> 800 IU vitamin E oil

Combine all of the ingredients. Apply two to four times per day with a glass rod or cotton swab to the warts only, since this is a very concentrated formula.

Menopause

Essential oils can help women get through menopause discomfort, such as hot flashes. Especially advantageous are essential oils that are thought to influence a woman's estrogen levels, such as clary sage and fennel. Geranium and lavender are hormonal balancers that modify menopause symptoms. Use them in a spray by adding 20 drops of essential oil to 2 ounces of distilled water in a spray bottle. Shake the mixture before using. Or try the essential oils in a bath, massage, or body oil.

▌Hormone-Balancing Essential Oils

Geranium   *Lavender*   *Neroli*

▌Estrogen-Enhancing Essential Oils

Clary sage   *Fennel*   *Sage*

Menopause Body Oil

If this formula is too oily for you, add these same essential oils to 4 ounces of a commercial body lotion instead of the vegetable oil. The best type to use is an unscented, basic lotion with all-natural ingredients.

    6 drops geranium

    3 drops clary sage

    2 drops peppermint (optional)

    2 drops fennel

    2 ounces vegetable oil

Combine all of the ingredients. Use daily as a body oil.

Hot Flash Spray

This formula could be made into smelling salts, but a spray is everyone's favorite choice when you need to cool down quickly. Clary sage works wonderfully, but you could also replace 6 drops of this formula with your favorite essential oil. Shake the bottle before using. Even spraying this as a room freshener does the trick, but your best bet is to close your eyes and spray your face.

    12 drops clary sage

    2 ounces water

Combine the ingredients in a spray bottle.

Vaginal Rejuvenation Oil

Neroli is an excellent essential oil to use, but if you find it too expensive, this formula can be made without it. The same essential oils can be added to 1 ounce of a commercial moisturizing cream or lubricant—just stir them in. Choose a product that is made with natural ingredients. To obtain the vitamin E, either purchase the liquid form or open capsules and empty the contents.

> 6 drops rose geranium
>
> 6 drops lavender
>
> 2 drops neroli (orange blossom)
>
> 1500 IU vitamin E oil
>
> 1 ounce vegetable oil

Combine all of the ingredients. Apply around and in the vagina as needed.

Muscle Cramps and PMS

Fortunately, essential oils can reduce painful muscle cramping, such as menstrual cramps. The same oils also help with PMS symptoms. Research shows some essential oils lower inflammatory hormonal substances like prostaglandins produced by the body that cause muscles to cramp and promote blood-sugar imbalance, headaches, nausea, breast tenderness and cysts, joint pain, water retention, moodiness, irritability, and even alcohol cravings. Try adding a few drops of the following oils to a long, relaxing bath or to massage oil.

Essential Oils to Relieve Cramps and PMS

Chamomile	*Frankincense*	*Marjoram*
Cinnamon	*Ginger*	*Melissa (lemon balm)*
Cloves	*Lavender*	*Thyme*

Cramp-Relieving Oil

This multipurpose oil can be used for all types of muscle spasms and cramps. Not only is this formula great for rubbing on the abdomen to relieve menstrual cramps, but it is also excellent for massaging onto the lower back to alleviate the aching that sometimes accompanies them.

> 12 drops lavender
>
> 6 drops marjoram
>
> 4 drops German chamomile
>
> 4 drops ginger
>
> 3 drops frankincense
>
> 2 ounces vegetable oil

Combine all of the ingredients and apply as often as needed over the cramping area.

Nerve and Joint Pain

I know people with serious nervous system problems, such as multiple sclerosis and chronic fatigue syndrome, who found pain relief by using a nerve pain oil. Although it may not offer a cure, it certainly improves quality of life. For carpal tunnel syndrome, rub this oil into the wrists. Use it on the back or hip for a pinched nerve or sciatica and on shingles to reduce pain. A number of essential oils, such as bergamot and cedarwood, have been shown to reduce physical pain just by sniffing them. Orange and lavender have successfully helped children overcome pain.

Essential Oils to Relieve Nerve and Joint Pain

Chamomile	*Lavender*	*Wintergreen or birch*
Frankincense	*Marjoram*	
Ginger	*Rosemary*	
Helichrysum	*Sandalwood*	

Nerve Pain Relief Oil

This is a concentrated formula, so rub it over just the painful area rather than using it as an all-body massage oil.

8 drops lavender

5 drops marjoram

2 drops frankincense

2 drops German chamomile

1 ounce vegetable oil

Combine all of the ingredients. Apply as needed for relief.

Arthritic Pain Oil

For arthritis, rheumatism, and similar inflammatory conditions, modify the nerve pain formula (opposite) by adding birch, which provides the same aroma and pain relief as wintergreen. I also like ginger for its anti-inflammatory properties and rosemary for its deep penetrating action.

> 4 drops wintergreen or birch
>
> 4 drops marjoram
>
> 3 drops lavender
>
> 3 drops rosemary
>
> 2 drops ginger
>
> 1 ounce vegetable oil

Combine all of the ingredients. Apply over painful or swollen areas as needed for relief.

Sinus and Respiratory Congestion

About 90 percent of respiratory ailments are caused by viruses. Fortunately, essential oils can inhibit viruses, including most of those responsible for flus and colds. Some oils even help loosen and eliminate lung and sinus congestion, making them excellent remedies for asthma and hay fever. Peppermint and eucalyptus reduce coughing and relax muscle spasms around the lungs.

Anyone who has ever sniffed eucalyptus or peppermint knows how well they clear the sinuses. Cypress dries up a persistent runny nose. *Caution:* Cinnamon and thyme are fine in a vapor balm or gargle, but steaming with them irritates the respiratory tract.

▌ Essential Oils to Relieve Congestion

Basil	*Eucalyptus*	*Peppermint*
Bay laurel	*Frankincense*	*Tea tree*
Cinnamon	*Ginger*	*Thyme*
Cypress	*Juniper*	

Aromatherapy Steam

Warm, moist steam opens nasal and bronchial passages, making it easier to breathe, and carries the essential oils to sinuses and lungs. Essential oils can be used in a humidifier or in a pan of water over low heat to disinfect the air. Lavender and eucalyptus are the most popular essential oils for sinus and lung steams. Studies show they are also some of the most effective general antibacterial, antiviral, and antifungal oils.

3 cups water

3 to 6 drops essential oils, such as eucalyptus or peppermint

Bring the water to a simmer in a pan. Remove the pan from the heat and add the essential oils. Place a towel over the back of your head, and tuck the ends around the pot so the steam is captured inside the improvised "tent." Take deep breaths of the steam for as long as is comfortable, then come out for air. Repeat this several times.

Homemade Nasal Inhaler

When steaming is impractical, use a natural nasal inhaler. You can buy one in natural-food stores or make your own with the following formula. The technique described in this formula can be used with any safe essential oil.

> ¼ teaspoon coarse salt
>
> 5 drops eucalyptus

Place the salt in a small vial (glass is best) with a tight-fitting lid, and add the eucalyptus oil. The salt will absorb the oil and provide a convenient way of carrying the oil without spilling it. When needed, open the vial and inhale deeply.

Vapor Rub

Vapor balms that are rubbed on the chest increase circulation and thus warm the body while they fight infection.

> 12 drops eucalyptus
>
> 5 drops peppermint
>
> 2 drops thyme
>
> 1 ounce olive oil

Combine all of the ingredients in a glass bottle. Shake well to mix the oils evenly. Gently massage into chest and throat.

Throat Spray/Gargle

An aromatherapy throat spray or gargle brings essential oils into direct contact with a sore throat or laryngitis. This versatile formula can be used both ways. At home, you can gargle with it. If you are at work or traveling, you'll find it more convenient to use it as a spray (to avoid spoilage, be sure to clean the spray bottle very well before adding the formula). You can find glycerin at drug and natural-food stores.

> 3 drops lemon
>
> 2 drops thyme
>
> ½ cup distilled water
>
> ½ teaspoon salt
>
> ½ teaspoon glycerin

Combine all of the ingredients in a lidded glass jar. Shake well to disperse the oils before using. Gargle a small amount throughout the day or pour it into a spray bottle and spray toward the back of the throat.

Varicose Veins and Hemorrhoids

The medical world offers patients little hope of recovery from varicose veins except through surgery. Essential oil products can reduce the size of varicose veins and hemorrhoids (a type of varicose vein) and ease the inflammation and pain they cause. They are especially effective when combined with exercise, an improved diet, and herbs that promote circulation.

Essential Oils to Relieve Varicose Veins and Hemorrhoids

Carrot seed   *German chamomile*   *Myrtle*

Cypress   *Helichrysum*   *Palmarosa*

Frankincense   *Lavender*

Varicose Vein and Hemorrhoid Formula

This formula works very well and even better if you use St. John's wort–infused herbal oil—which you can buy in a natural-food store or make yourself (see page 30)—as a base instead of the vegetable oil.

6 drops cypress

3 drops myrtle

3 drops German chamomile

2 drops frankincense

1 ounce vegetable oil

Combine all of the ingredients. Apply externally.

Carrot Seed Compress

When varicose veins become severe, the skin may be ulcerated and broken. If this occurs, apply this compress for relief.

> 4 drops lavender
>
> 8 drops carrot seed
>
> ½ cup water

Add the essential oils to the water. Slosh a soft cloth in the water, wring it out, fold it, and place it over ulcerated veins.

MOTHER AND
BABY CARE

For pregnant women and young children, use only the gentlest essential oils and reduce the amount in formulas to one-third. Be cautious using any essential oils during the first trimester of pregnancy, especially if prone to miscarriage. Massage and aromatherapy both help prevent stretch marks from forming as a pregnant belly expands. Apply belly oil twice a day. Lavender is one of the gentlest essential oils and keeps skin supple. It is an old companion in the birthing room. Many women appreciate a relaxing lavender massage during labor. In the days following childbirth, sniffing clary sage helps counter postpartum depression.

Gentle Essential Oils for Mother and Baby

Chamomile	*Jasmine*	*Rose*
Frankincense	*Lavender*	*Sandalwood*
Geranium	*Neroli*	*Spearmint*

Diaper Rash

Aromatherapy baby oil and powder protect your baby from diaper rash. The oil forms a barrier on the skin that repels moisture; the powder absorbs moisture and prevents chafing. Use them every diaper change. The oil is also excellent for baby massage. Avoid commercial, petroleum-based baby oils made from mineral oil, which is questionable for skin use. Pure cornstarch alternatives are a better choice than powders containing talc.

Pregnant Belly Oil

You can rub your own belly—or better yet, get someone to do it for you! Obtain vitamin E by pricking open a few capsules or buying it as a liquid.

> ½ ounce cocoa butter
>
> 4 ounces vegetable oil
>
> 12 drops (⅛ teaspoon) lavender
>
> 5 drops neroli or rose (expensive, so optional)
>
> 1600 IU vitamin E

In a pan over very low heat, melt the cocoa butter in the vegetable oil. Remove the pan from the heat. Stir in the essential oils and vitamin E, and pour the mixture into a glass bottle. Massage your belly with the oil at least a couple times daily.

Herbal Baby Oil

Baby oil needs to be very dilute so even these gentle oils do not irritate baby's sensitive skin. Do not use it on genitals or face. Do not use any aromatherapy on the skin of newborns.

> 12 drops lavender
>
> 4 drops German chamomile
>
> 4 ounces vegetable oil

Combine all of the ingredients.

Fragrant Baby Powder

Spice or salt shakers with large perforations in the lid make good powder dispensers for this powder.

4 ounces cornstarch

12 drops lavender

Put the cornstarch in a zip-top plastic bag and drop or spray in the essential oil using a glass spray bottle. Tightly close the bag and toss back and forth to distribute the oil, breaking up any clumps by pressing them with your fingers through the bag. Let stand for at least 4 days, continuing to break up the clumps. Pour into a shaker and use each time you change a diaper.

Bread feeds the body, indeed, but flowers feed the soul.
—THE KORAN

Teething Oil

Clove teething oil has been popular for a long time. However, it can burn the gums. Try it on your own gums, and you will see how it will burn the more sensitive mouth of an infant. Chamomile is slightly less effective as a pain reliever, but it is not as hot as the clove. Remember to dilute any essential oil before putting it on the gums.

> 1 drop German chamomile or 1 drop clove bud
>
> 1 tablespoon vegetable oil

Combine the ingredients. Rub a few drops on painful gums. Repeat every hour or so.

HOME
IMPROVEMENTS

Essential oils can keep your house smelling fresh. They are also natural repellents to keep away pesky insects such as mosquitoes and moths. It's easy to make your own potpourris, room fresheners, and bug repellents.

Scenting a Room

Fragrance positively affects the emotions of everyone in a room and disinfects airborne bacteria.

Air Fresheners

A popular way to scent a room is a plug-in that goes directly into an electrical outlet. Rather than purchasing a plug-in scented with synthetic fragrance, choose one with unscented pads that you scent yourself with natural oils. Another method is to place three to six drops of an essential oil into a pan of gently steaming water on the stove. Electric and candle-heated potpourri cookers have a small bowl where you place a few essential oil drops in a small amount of water.

Quite a selection of electric diffusers are available in many attractive designs. Add your choice of essential oils to them and they disperse the scent throughout a room. Some diffusers release the fragrance via steam. There are even ones that can be set as an alarm clock to wake you with a burst of aroma.

Modern potpourris owe most of their fragrance to essential oils that are added to an attractive collection of dried herbs. They make lovely room fresheners when set around the house.

For a stronger room freshener, use an aromatherapy spray (20 drops essential oil per 2 ounces distilled water, shaken). You can also spray room disinfectant in a sickroom or use it on a kitchen counter. I know one mom who sprays the kids' bedrooms every evening with a soothing chamomile and ylang-ylang mix.

Disinfectant Room Spray and Natural Cleanser

Keep this spray in a spritzer bottle, which can be found in most drugstores and in some cosmetics stores.

> 4 drops eucalyptus or tea tree
>
> 3 drops lavender
>
> 2 drops bergamot
>
> 2 drops thyme
>
> 1 drop peppermint
>
> 2 ounces distilled water

Add the essential oils to the water and pour into a spritzer bottle. Shake well right before each use, as some of the oil will float on the surface.

Scented Items

You can scent cloth, except for silk and delicate fabrics that stain. Use an aromatherapy spray to disperse the scent on pillows, bed linens, and clothes. To scent paper products like stationery, add a few drops of essential oil to a piece of paper, and place it in a plastic bag along with the items you wish to scent. After a couple days, the fragrance will have lightly permeated the contents.

Potpourri

Potpourri is a mixture of fragrant, dried plants. It is kept in a closed container in an easy-to-reach location so the lid can be lifted off and the fragrance enjoyed or in an open container to dissipate the scent into a small area of a room. Potpourri can also be placed in a porous bag that releases its scent into the air. The scented herbs that fill the sleep pillow on page 51 are potpourri. Turn any potpourri into an aromatherapy experience by choosing dried herbs that have significant healing properties. Essential oils are often added directly to the herb or the container to increase the scent.

There are several essential oil fixatives that make the scent of potpourri last for many years, including patchouli, sandalwood, benzoin, clary sage, balsam of Peru, balsam of tolu, and vetiver. The violet-scented orris root powder is the traditional potpourri preservative, although a number of people are allergic to orris, so its use has declined. Its light scent blends with almost any fragrance. An orris essential oil for perfumes is rare and costly, so I use the root instead. For the potpourri's dried plant material, use your favorite combination of attractive flowers, leaves, or cones.

> 1 cup dried plant material
>
> 1 tablespoon orris root,
> finely chopped (optional)
>
> ¼ teaspoon essential oil (your choice)

Place the dried plant material in a closable container, then add the orris root, if desired. Using an eyedropper, drop the essential oil onto the orris root, making sure it is dispersed throughout. (If you do not use orris root,

continued

drop the essential oil directly onto the potpourri.) Keep in the closed container for several days—enough time for the scent to permeate the plant material—then transfer into an open display container. This potpourri should stay fragrant for many months. When it gets faint, revive it with a few drops of essential oil. For a potpourri to be simmered on the stovetop, double the quantity of essential oil, using ½ teaspoon per cup of dried plant material.

Bug Repellent

I will not claim that aromatherapy bug repellents work better than drugstore varieties, but they are a good alternative to toxic chemicals. Mosquitoes, ticks, and many other outdoor insect pests hate pungent essential oils such as citronella; unfortunately, so do quite a few people. Your bug repellent will be more fragrant if you add geranium. Reduce the insect population outdoors with citronella candles that release the scent as they burn. Peppermint serves as an all-around insect repellent for both indoors and your garden, repelling ants and aphids.

Natural Mosquito Repellents

Cedarwood	*Eucalyptus*	*Pennyroyal*
Citronella	*Geranium*	

Bug Repellent

This repellent will last for at least a year. Be sure not to rub your eyes right after applying it to your skin with your fingers; the oils will irritate them.

¼ teaspoon citronella

¼ teaspoon eucalyptus

⅛ teaspoon cedarwood

⅛ teaspoon geranium

2 ounces carrier oil or alcohol

Combine all of the ingredients. Store in a glass bottle.

Citronella Candle

Why buy expensive store-bought candles when you can make your own naturally scented ones?

20 drops citronella

Votive candle, unscented

Using a glass dropper, drip the oil onto the candle's unlit wick. Give the wick 24 hours to absorb the oil before the candle is ready to burn.

Peppermint Bug Spray

In this spray, the soap helps the oil combine with the water.

> ½ teaspoon peppermint oil
>
> ½ cup water
>
> 1 tablespoon liquid dish or hand soap

Combine all of the ingredients in a spray bottle and shake before using.

---

*To comfort the braine, smel to chamomile,
eate sage . . . wash measurably, sleep reasonably,
delight to heare melody and singing.*

—RAMS LITTLE DODOEN,
SEVENTEENTH-CENTURY HERBAL

Moth Repellent

The traditional way to keep moths out of your woolens is to store them in a cedarwood or camphor chest. In India, patchouli keeps moths out of Oriental carpets—in fact, when Europeans started producing cheaper imitations of these rugs, wary buyers knew they were not authentic because they did not smell like patchouli. Modern mothballs are harsh, displeasing imitations of camphor; worse, they are toxic. It is far better to use a pleasant-smelling, natural alternative.

▌ Moth Repellents

Cedarwood *Patchouli* *Tansy*

Lavender *Sage* *Wormwood*

Natural Wool-Moth Repellent

For more attractive mothballs, tie a small fabric square around each cotton ball.

20 drops cedarwood

8 drops lavender

8 drops patchouli or sage

1 dozen cotton balls

Combine the essential oils and place 3 drops on each cotton ball. Store in a closed container for a couple of days. Place with clothes, using about six balls for an average-size box or suitcase.

Flea Control

When you have a flea infestation, each day vacuum areas where your pet spends time, then spray the area with a cedar-wood repellent. Do not put products containing essential oils directly on your pet's fur or skin or use collars saturated with essential oils. Despite all the essential oil products on the market, dogs and especially cats do not have the proper liver enzymes to break down and process essential oils. Instead, essential oils build up in their systems and poison them. There are many reports of animals going into comas, experiencing liver failure, and even dying from essential oils. Just because a pet does not show any visual signs of being harmed by oils does not mean there's no internal damage. An additional problem with cats is that they continually lick their coats and ingest oils on their fur. Cats have even been injured from inhaling the air in a room with an essential oil diffuser that is on constantly.

Use flea-repelling essential oils to create a spray to spray or the ground herbs to powder around areas where pets hang out. However, be aware that your pet will not appreciate this gesture since animals usually dislike the smell of essential oils.

Flea Repellents

Bay laurel   *Citronella*   *Lemon*

Cedarwood   *Eucalyptus*   *Pennyroyal*

Cedarwood Spray

This spray is very effective for flea-infested carpets, and it smells great, too.

1 cup water

20 drops cedarwood

Mix together in a spray bottle. Because essential oils and water do not mix easily, shake well before each spray.

Flea Powder

Do not apply this repellent powder directly to fur since the animal may lick it off.

> **20 drops cedarwood**
>
> **1 cup cornstarch**

Add the essential oil to the cornstarch and stir to distribute. Let the mixture sit for a few days, enough time for the oil to dissipate through the cornstarch. Sprinkle on rugs and carpets. Sprinkle lightly on dog beds. Do not apply to areas where cats sleep.

MATERIA MEDICA:
COMMON
ESSENTIAL OILS

Basil *Ocimum basilicum*

Distilled from the leaves and flowering tops, this familiar sweet-and-spicy kitchen herb reduces stress, rattled nerves, anxiety, and anger. A sixteenth-century basil cologne was considered a mood enhancer. Japanese researchers found the aroma stimulates the brain's beta waves to increase alertness and reduce fatigue. Basil relieves headaches, sinus congestion, temporary loss of the sense of smell, nausea (even from chemotherapy), indigestion, and sore muscles. It treats viral and fungal infection and the herpes and shingles viruses. It helps both oily and problem complexions.

Bay Laurel *Laurus nobilis*

The pungent, spicy aroma distilled from the leaves of this tree sharpens the wit; hence, the ancient Greeks placed bay wreaths on the heads of scholars and athletes. They also used it for its reputation for enhancing memory. The Greek priestesses at Delphi sat over burning bay fumes to induce prophetic visions. A massage oil containing bay stimulates lymph and circulation and helps with sinus and lung congestion. "Bay" cologne and soap is made with the spicier bay rum (*Pimenta racemosa*), which can irritate mucous membranes.

Bergamot *Citrus bergamia*

The fresh, clean scent comes from the cold-pressed rind of this small green citrus fruit. It counters depression, anxiety, insomnia, and stress. Some say it even helps with compulsive behavior, including eating disorders. Researchers found that the aroma can reduce the sensations of pain. Named after Bergamo, Italy, where the tree originated, the essential oil scents colognes and flavors Earl Grey tea and some candies. Bergamot kills fungal infection and several viruses—including flu, herpes, shingles, and chickenpox—and reduces mouth, throat, and skin inflammation and infection. It also aids the immune system. It is used on oily complexions. *Note:* The essential oil contains the photosensitizing bergapten compound. Bergapten-free oil is available. Do not confuse it with garden bergamot or bee balm (*Monarda didyma*).

Carrot Seed *Daucus carota*

A sharp, pungent essential oil is distilled from the seeds of wild carrot, an ancestor of our garden carrot. It benefits oily and problem complexions. It enhances skin tone and elasticity and decreases dryness, wrinkles, dermatitis, eczema, rashes, and even some precancerous skin conditions. It also stimulates circulation and treats various reproductive system and digestive disorders.

Cedarwood *Cedrus* spp.

The soft, woodsy fragrance of this tree's wood and needles is distilled into an essential oil that often scents soap and cologne. It is used to enhance stability, meditation, and intuition, while relieving stress and aggression. Researchers found that simply smelling the aroma can reduce the sensations of pain. Use it on oily skin and scalp, dandruff, dermatitis, bites, and itchy skin. A massage oil can be rubbed over the area to treat respiratory and bladder infections. Cedarwood repels insects such as wool moths. The legendary "cedar of Lebanon" Moroccan cedarwood (*C. libani*) was prized by ancient cultures. Atlas cedarwood (*C. atlantica*) is from Morocco. The warm and almost spicy Himalayan cedarwood (*C. deodara*) is the least harsh on skin, although there are concerns about it being overharvested.

Chamomile, German
Matricaria recutita; M. chamomilla

The sweet, herbaceous, and applelike aroma distilled from chamomile's flowers reduces stress, insomnia, and PMS and helps to calm fussy babies, according to several studies. Used externally, it relieves the inflammation and discomfort of headaches, skin rashes, allergies, enlarged veins, and sore muscles, tendons, and joints, as well as nerve and menstrual pain. Chamomile is a stronger pain reliever than most people realize. In several studies, it worked as well as pharmaceutical drugs to ease pain during painful hospital procedures—in one case when patients simply smelled it. It also treats indigestion and boosts immunity. It is excellent for any skin type, with dry or problem skin conditions its specialty. The more anti-inflammatory German chamomile is blue, whereas Roman chamomile (*Chamaemelum nobile; Anthemis nobilis*) is pale yellow. The scent of either one helps to overcome anxiety, depression, and hyperactivity. *Note:* Sometimes sold as "blue chamomile" are ormensis (*Ormensis multicaulis*), tansy (*Tanacetum annuum*), and wormwood (*Artemisia arborescens*). The last two essential oils are potentially toxic, so they are rarely used in aromatherapy.

Cinnamon *Cinnamomum zeylanicum*

Distilled from the tree's leaf or bark, cinnamon has a sweet, spicy-hot fragrance. It relieves tension but still invigorates the senses and is stimulating, decreasing fatigue. It was a popular Indian and European aphrodisiac. Small amounts still spice up Oriental perfume blends. It improves digestion, blood vessel integrity, and the immune system. An antioxidant, antiviral, and antifungal, it helps preserve aromatherapy products. It adds heat to liniments to reduce muscle pain and menstrual cramps. Use it in very small amounts because it is hot enough to irritate and even burn skin. *Note:* Cassia, or *kuei pi* (*C. cassia*), is an inexpensive substitute from China used in medicine, seasoning, incense, and drinks.

Citronella *Citronella nardus*

Citronella is a grasslike plant, and the sharp lemon scent of its inexpensive essential oil is found in many cleaning products. The most popular use of the distilled essential oil is to ward off insects, especially mosquitoes. Citronella also treats colds, infections, and an oily complexion. It often adulterates the far more expensive lemon verbena and melissa (lemon balm) oils, although it smells far sharper and more camphoric and can irritate the skin.

Clary Sage *Salvia sclarea*

Distilled from the herb's flowering tops and leaves, clary's scent is an intense blend of sweet, pungent, and heady aromas. It is relaxing and euphoric and enhances dreams. It counters panic, paranoia, stress, and mental fatigue. Clary sage was once recommended to increase joy, and research suggests that it acts on brain receptors as an antidepressant, maybe even more than lavender or German chamomile. But sniffing too much can have a hypnotic effect. It eases PMS, postpartum depression, and menopause problems such as hot flashes probably because it slightly stimulates estrogen and the adrenal glands. Researchers have suggested it to relax women who are undergoing stressful medical procedures. Clary sage eases muscle and nervous tension, pain, and muscle cramps. It helps rejuvenate hair and any skin type, but especially mature, problem, or inflamed skin and reduces dandruff. *Note:* Although clary is related to culinary sage (*Salvia officinalis*), its actions are quite different. Culinary sage essential oil concentrates thujone, which is potentially neurotoxic, so use it carefully and not around anyone prone to seizures. The small amount of garden sage used in cooking presents no problem.

Clove Bud
Syzygium aromaticum; Eugenia caryophyllata
The spicy, hot scent is distilled from the immature buds, leaves, or stems of the clove tree. It may be spicy, but the scent is relaxing, helping to overcome nervousness, stress, mental fatigue, and poor memory. It is also sometimes used as an antidepressant aroma. When greatly diluted, it sweetens the breath and dulls toothache pain. It also treats flu, sore muscles, arthritis, colds, and bronchial congestion and is used to heat up liniments. The eugenol compound from clove is made into drugs that kill germs and relieve pain. As a mouthwash, it eliminates the *Helicobacter pylori* bacteria that lingers in the mouth and is responsible for stomach ulcers. A potent antioxidant, clove is being studied for its ability to protect cells from some types of cancer. It is also an antifungal. Avoid using the leaf, which can irritate skin and mucous membranes.

Cypress *Cupressus sempervirens*
Distilled from the needles, twigs, or cones of the tree, the sharp, pungent, pinelike, spicy scent of cypress is common in men's aftershave. It eases grief and sometimes insomnia, although the scent can sometimes be stimulating. Studies show that the aroma can reduce the sensations of pain. The smoke was inhaled in southern Europe to relieve sinus

and lung congestion; the Chinese chewed the small cones to reduce gum inflammation. The massage oil helps with circulatory problems, such as low blood pressure, varicose veins, hemorrhoids, and cellulite. Cypress also alleviates laryngitis. In skin care, it is used on oily skin. As a deodorant, it reduces excessive sweating. *Note:* Do not confuse it with the anti-inflammatory essential oil of Hinoki cypress (*Chamaecyparis obtusa*).

Eucalyptus *Eucalyptus globulus*

Distilled from leaves and twigs, eucalyptus essential oil has a distinctive pungent, sharp, and camphoric fragrance that increases mental energy and is stimulating enough to help keep you awake. The essential oil (or its component eucalyptol) is used in commercial aftershave, cologne, mouthwash, liniments, and chest rubs. It is a potent antiviral, antibacterial, and antifungal that also aids the immune system. Use it in massage oil or salve or to treat sinus, throat, herpes, and lung infections. It is excellent on an oily complexion—especially one with acne—as well as boils and insect bites. The essential oil comes in several species, varieties, and chemotypes. Aromatherapists often prefer the chemotype of a different species called blue malle (*Eucalyptus polybractea* ct. *cineol*) for treating sinus and bronchial congestion.

Fennel *Foeniculum vulgare*

This essential oil, distilled from the seeds, has an herbaceous, sweet, and licorice-like scent. Inhaling it has been found to stimulate the nervous system and apparently the pituitary, adrenal, and hypothalamus glands to reduce stress and its negative impact. The aroma is used for self-motivation and to counter fatigue. Historically, it has represented strength and longevity. Fennel helps with obesity, water retention, urinary tract problems, and indigestion. Its hormonal properties influence estrogen to increase mother's milk. It refines the mature complexion and heals bruises. *Note:* Large amounts can overexcite the nervous system. Do not use with anyone who has nervous system problems or epilepsy.

Fir *Abies alba*

The woodsy, sharp essential oil is distilled from the twigs or needles. It commonly comes from *Abies alba*, but several different fir tree species are distilled. The aroma is said to enhance intuition and the sense of being both grounded and elevated. Fir in massage oil soothes muscle and rheumatism pain, increases poor circulation, and inhibits bronchial infections and coughing. It is also used to treat skin infections.

Frankincense *Boswellia carterii*

This small gnarly tree grows on the rocky hillsides of Yemen, Oman, and Somalia. When distilled, the oleo gum resin produces a soft balsamic essential oil that is relaxing, slowing and deepening breathing. For ages, it has soothed the spirit and enhanced perception, meditation, and prayer. It is sometimes used to dispel grief. Use it externally on mature or dry skin, acne, fungal infections, boils, hard-to-heal wounds, and scars. Frankincense also treats the lungs and relieves congestion. Studies show the less expensive and aromatic Indian frankincense (*Boswellia serrata*) that is available in drugstores as Boswellia cream relieves muscle, joint, and nerve pain and inflammation.

Geranium, Rose *Pelargonium graveolens*

Also known simply as *geranium*, the oil is distilled from the leaves to create a rosy, citrusy, woodsy, and herbal aromatic combination that relieves anxiety, depression, stress, anger, and mood swings. Although regarded as sedative, it is a light adrenal-gland stimulant that may help balance hormones. Simply taking a sniff helps with PMS, menopause, and blood pressure. Suitable for most skin types, it reduces inflammation; bacterial, fungal, and viral infections; eczema; acne; herpes; ringworm; scarring; and stretch marks.

Ginger *Zingiber officinale*

Distilled from the rhizome, ginger's spicy, warm, and sharp fragrance adds a nice touch to formulas. It has both a stimulating and an aphrodisiac effect. It helps heat up a warming liniment to relieve muscle, joint, and nerve pain. The massage oil treats appetite loss, nausea, inflammation, and lung infection. Just sniffing the scent relieves nausea. It relieves sinus congestion.

Helichrysum *Helichrysum angustifolium*

A pleasant spicy, currylike fragrance is distilled from the flowers of this herb, sometimes called everlasting or *immortelle*. This aroma is one of the most potent scents on the brain's GABA neurotransmitter receptors to alleviate depression, stress, and burnout. The essential oil reduces bronchitis and inflammation from muscle or nerve pain or arthritis. It counters allergic reactions like asthma. It also appears to stimulate new cell production. Helichrysum creams and lotions are used on acne, scar tissue, bruises, burns, varicose veins, and couperose or mature skin.

Jasmine *Jasminum officinale; J. grandiflorum*

An absolute and a concrete (see glossary) are made from jasmine's blossoms. The complex floral and sweetly exotic fragrance is found in expensive perfume. It increases pleasant emotions, mental accuracy, vigilance, and visual awareness; overcomes insomnia and depression; and takes the edge off anger. The uplifting fragrance is stimulating—it sometimes slightly raises breathing rate and blood pressure—slightly hypnotic, and definitely aphrodisiac. It also reduces mental and physical fatigue. Its Iranian name even means "heavenly joy." It eases headaches and menstrual cramps. It is good for sensitive, dry, and mature complexions. The most prized oil comes from France and Italy, although most is from Egypt.

Juniper *Juniperus communis*

The berries of this North American shrub are distilled into higher-quality essential oil than the needles and branches. The scent of the berries is pungent, herbaceous, and peppery. A sedative component in the essential oil called cedrol is suggested to counter anxiety and stress and can even work to reduce fatigue. The branches have been burned in the Mediterranean and southwest China as well as by some western North American indigenous tribes for purification, protection, and warding off contagious disease during healing ceremonies. Juniper massage oil or salve treats rheumatic pain, general debility, varicose veins, hemorrhoids, fluid retention, cellulite, and bronchial infections and congestion. It is also antiviral and an excellent antiseptic and wound healer. Research found it helps with indigestion and is particularly potent in stopping foot odor and destroying the bacteria that causes it. Juniper is suitable in cosmetics for acne, eczema, oily hair, and dandruff. There has been discussion that juniper overstimulates inflamed kidneys, but at least one study says that is not so. For bladder infections, rub it in a massage oil over the area.

Lavender *Lavandula angustifolia*

Distilled from the herb's flower buds, lavender's sweetly floral aroma is also herbal, with balsamic undertones. It is specifically used for problems associated with the central nervous system; and studies back it to treat a variety of emotional problems such as nervousness, exhaustion, insomnia, irritability, stress, anxiety, and depression. It is used to help increase focus and concentration while maintaining little stress. The essential oil relieves pain and inflammation, such as that from tight muscles, headaches, insect bites, rashes, bruises, and skin infections. A skin-cell regenerator, it is suitable for all complexion types, diminishing scarring, stretch marks, wrinkles, burns, and sun damage. It helps with lung and sinus infections, eases indigestion, and boosts immunity. One-half drop per suppository helps get rid of vaginal infections, including candida.

Lemon *Citrus limonum*

Pressed from the fresh peel, lemon essential oil is an antidepressant that has long been said to create a feeling of "cleansing" the emotions. It is an antioxidant, a preservative, and an antiseptic used to reverse viral and bacterial infections and boost immunity. As massage oil, it is useful for easing high blood pressure, congested lymph glands, and water retention. Use it in formulas for oily complexions. *Note:* Lemon essential oil can cause skin photosensitivity—a temporary rash when going out in the sun—for a few people.

Lemongrass *Cymbopogon citratus*

This lemon-herby fragrance is sedative and soothing with antidepressant properties similar to lemon. The essential oil, distilled from its grasslike leaves, scents cosmetics, deodorants, and soaps, including the classic Ivory brand. In massage oil, it treats the pain of indigestion, rheumatism, and headaches. Researchers think it helps keep blood vessels open by toning their lining. It is suggested for oily hair; acne; bacterial, viral, and fungal skin infections; and ringworm. *Note:* Lemongrass is nontoxic, but it does produce a skin reaction in a few people who are sensitive to it.

Lemon Verbena *Aloysia triphylla*

The essential oil, distilled from the lemon-scented leaves, has a very soothing effect on both the mind and body. The pleasant scent encourages relaxation and sleep and eases nervous indigestion and depression. Sniffing it also aids in concentration and focus. It can be used as a steam or chest rub to treat colds, lung congestion, and asthma. The essential oil is excellent as hair rinse and in products designed for normal or oily complexions.

Marjoram
Origanum marjorana; Marjorana hortensis

Distilled from the leaves of the culinary herb, the sweet yet herbal, sharp aroma hints of camphor and helps with emotional instability, debility, irritability, stress, anxiety, and even hysteria. It is a potent antidepressant. Historically, it eased loneliness, a broken heart, and grief. This sedative aroma relieves headaches and high blood pressure. Studies suggest inhaling the scent to reduce stress and to fall asleep more easily. The body oil eases muscle spasms, menstrual cramps, nerve pain, stiff joints, and spasmodic coughing. It also counters indigestion, colds, flu, and laryngitis. Use it on the skin to tend bruises, burns, inflammation, and fungal and bacterial infections. Marjoram is safer and less harsh on the skin than its relative oregano.

Melissa (Lemon Balm) *Melissa officinalis*

Distilled from the leaves of lemon balm, melissa's sweet smell is soft and lemony. Shock, distress, stress, depression, anxiety, nervousness, and insomnia are helped by its sedative properties. Melissa was the main ingredient in "Carmelite water" complexion toner made by Carmelite nuns in the Middle Ages to counter skin inflammation and fungal and viral infections such as herpes. In massage oil, it is suggested for treating indigestion, lung congestion, strep throat, high blood pressure, and menstrual problems. *Note:* Not easily distilled, this expensive oil is often adulterated with lemon, citronella, or even lemon eucalyptus.

Myrrh *Commiphora myrrha*

The tree gum is distilled into a warm, resinous oil. The scent of both oil and incense containing myrrh has been used since antiquity to inspire prayer and meditation and to fortify the spirit. It has a history of being sedative and is used to relieve stress and promote relaxation. Studies show that the fragrance of a low-grade type of myrrh called opopanax (*Commiphora erythraea*) does relax the nervous system. Myrrh helps with coughs and immunity. It treats wounds, gum disease, chapped or aged skin, eczema, bruises, skin infections, varicose veins, and fungal infections.

Neroli (Orange Blossom)
Citrus aurantium var. amara

This sweet and intensely heady fragrance is distilled from the blossoms of the bitter orange tree. One of the best aromatic antidepressants, it counters emotional shock, confusion, nervousness, anxiety, depression, fear, fatigue, and insomnia. The aroma slightly lowers high blood pressure. It is used on mature and couperose skin to regenerate cells.

Orange Citrus sinensis

Cold-pressed from the sweet orange peel, this familiar scent is lively. A sedative fragrance, it helps during depression, anxiety, shock, and nervous tension. Studies back its use to relieve pain—just by smell alone—and to help during stressful situations. It even slightly lowers high blood pressure. Orange treats flu, colds, and congested lymph. It is sometimes used on oily complexions, although it can be photosensitizing to skin. Tangerine and mandarin (*Citrus reticulata*) have similar properties.

Palmarosa Cymbopogon martini

The lemon-rose fragrance of this grass is reminiscent of the richer and more expensive rose geranium, which it sometimes replaces. Distilled from its grasslike leaves, the aroma has been shown to treat stress and nervous exhaustion in studies. Its traditional use is to treat disorders related to the nervous system, such as epilepsy and pain. A cell regenerator, it balances oil production of any complexion type, but especially dry, acne, or infected skin.

Patchouli *Pogostemon cablin*

Distilled from aged, fermented leaves, the heavy, earthy, and musty aroma of patchouli dissipates nervousness and emotional exhaustion. It has long been considered an aphrodisiac in its native India. It is an antidepressant, except to those who dislike the scent! Patchouli reduces appetite and water retention and also counters flu and inflammation. As an antiseptic cell rejuvenator, it treats acne, eczema, athlete's foot, cracked or mature skin, dandruff, and inflammation, such as bruises and rashes.

Pepper, Black *Piper nigrum*

The distilled oil comes from the partly dried, unripe fruit—the same pepper we sprinkle on food. The spicy, sharp scent is invigorating and, some say, aphrodisiac. Pepper treats colds, flu, bladder infections, congested lungs, fevers, and poor circulation—typically in a body oil. Though nontoxic and not as hot as peppercorns, the oil sometimes irritates skin.

Peppermint *Mentha x piperita*

Distilled from the leaves of the herb, the powerful, fresh aroma combines the scents of pepper and mint. Studies show that inhaling peppermint for thirty seconds every five minutes improves memory, mood, accuracy, visual perception, and vigilance. The strong scent also counters shock and is sometimes used to reverse anxiety. Peppermint relieves muscle spasms, inflammation, nausea, and sinus and lung congestion. Well known for easing digestive problems, it also destroys bacteria, viruses, and parasites in the digestive tract. Enteric capsules of peppermint are designed to treat irritable bowel syndrome by not releasing essential oil until they reach the bowel. Studies show that it improves exercise performance, breath capacity, and lung tone. Small amounts of the essential oil in a cream or salve stimulate oil production on dry skin and relieve itching from ringworm, herpes, and poison oak and ivy. Peppermint is in most liniments to increase the sensation of heat by creating a hot/cold effect on the skin.

Petitgrain *Citrus aurantium*
Now distilled from the leaves and stems of the bitter orange tree, this oil originally came from the unripe fruit, hence the name, which means "little fruit." Petitgrain's aroma resembles neroli, which is produced from the flowers of the same species, but it is more herby, sharper, and less expensive. Like many citrus scents, it is an antidepressant that also helps to reduce anxiety, stress, and insomnia.

Rose *Rosa damascena*, and other species
This costly oil is distilled, or solvent extracted, from the blossoms. The divine, relaxing fragrance helps in depression, anxiety, grief, and lack of confidence. It has long represented spirituality, love, and an open heart that makes one more receptive as well as being aphrodisiac. The buds have been crafted into fragrant prayer beads. It appears to relieve stress and help with insomnia by working through the brain's hypothalamus and pituitary gland and by activating the neurotransmitter GABA. Research shows that smelling roses relaxes emotional and physical tension through the sympathetic nervous system. It reduces pain as much as 40 percent, sometimes as well as pharmaceutical drugs. Rose may even provide an adjunct therapy for morphine addiction. A cell rejuvenator with a reputation for slowing the skin's aging, rose soothes and heals all skin conditions

and complexion types. As an antiseptic, it fights skin and lung infections and digestive problems.

Rosemary *Rosmarinus officinalis*

This aroma, distilled from the herb's flowering tops, smells herbal, sharp, and camphoric. Research shows the stimulating scent helps reduce fatigue, tension, anxiety, and confusion. Inhaling rosemary activates the brain's beta waves to decrease levels of the primary stress hormone, cortisol, in just five minutes. Rosemary's cineole compound slows the breakdown of a neurotransmitter involved in memory and other mental processes. Sprigs were once worn in the hair and the smoke inhaled to counteract "brain weakness" and enhance spiritual awareness. They were also worn by brides and carried at funerals to represent remembrance of the ancestors. Rosemary's scent was considered helpful to resolve grief. It also eases dizziness and nightmares and encourages dream recall. The massage oil helps with poor circulation, sore muscles, nerve pain, rheumatism, indigestion, and cellulite. It raises low blood pressure and treats high cholesterol, moving lymph, lung congestion, sore throat, and canker sores. Rosemary was the main ingredient in "Hungary Water," which served as a cologne, facial toner, and memory aid. Rosemary is antibacterial and antiviral, as well as a strong antioxidant and natural preservative. There are several rosemary chemotypes, such as the more gently scented verbenone type, which is recommended for dry and problem skin.

Sandalwood *Santalum album*

Distilled from the tree's heartwood or roots, this oil's scent is balsamic, soft, warm, and woody. Sandalwood counters inflammation, hemorrhoids, persistent coughs, nausea, throat problems, and nerve pain. Suitable for all complexion types, sandalwood is useful on rashes, inflammation, acne, and chapped skin. It also treats depression, anxiety, and insomnia and helps instill peaceful relaxation, openness, and a sense of grounding. It has long been used to enhance prayer and meditation. Look for sustainable sandalwood that is plantation grown.

Tea Tree *Melaleuca alternifolia*

This sharp-smelling oil distilled from the tree leaves has a medicinal aroma that is similar to eucalyptus. An energizing oil, it increases mental focus. Numerous studies back its use as an immune tonic and a strong antiseptic against lung, sinus, mouth, bladder, vaginal, and fungal infections, as well as viral infections such as herpes, shingles, chickenpox, candida, thrush, and flu. It also reduces lung and sinus congestion. There are several medicinal species varieties. "MQV" (*M. quinquenervia*), which has a slightly sweeter fragrance, is considered a stronger antiviral and anti-inflammatory. A massage oil treats diaper rash, acne, wounds, and insect bites and protects the skin from radiation burns caused by cancer therapy. It is excellent to treat oily skin and acne. It kills mites, ticks, and head lice. *Note:* Although touted as nonirritating, tea tree essential oil can irritate sensitive skin.

Thyme *Thymus vulgaris*

The scent, from distillation of the leaves and tiny flowers, is herbal, warm, and sharp. It relieves melancholy and nightmares and prevents memory loss. Italian research suggests that a main component, carvacrol, causes the brain's neurotransmitters to increase feelings of well-being and dismiss depression. The Scots drank wild thyme tea to inspire vigor and bravery. Thyme is a strong antibacterial and antiviral for mouth and lung infections, as well as an antifungal that also boosts the immune system. It relieves indigestion, coughs, and lung congestion and was once specific for whooping cough. It is used in heating liniments, but use it cautiously since it can blister skin. The many thyme chemotypes have slightly different scents and specific properties. The linalool type, which is not a skin irritant, is especially good to treat a problem complexion.

Vanilla *Vanilla planifolia*

The sweet, creamy scent—obtained as a resinoid, absolute, or oleoresin, or by CO_2 extraction—is consoling with a reputation for improving confidence and sensuality and relieving stress and anxiety. Psychoanalysts have used it to help bring back their patients' childhood memories. The true oil is expensive, so most "vanilla" essential oil on the market is actually synthetic. The scent of vanilla extract from the grocery store is inexpensive and has the same properties, although it has a water-soluble base, so it cannot be mixed into vegetable oil carriers.

Vetiver
Chrysopogon zizanioides; Vetiveria zizanioides

Distilled from the roots, the earthy and heavy scent is called "oil of tranquility" in India, where it is recommended for nervousness, oversensitivity, and cooling down anger. In India and Indonesia, window screens called *tatties* woven from vetiver roots are sprinkled with water on hot days to scent and cool the house. Research suggests vetiver stimulates the nervous system, improving reaction times, the ability to quickly differentiate objects, and computer work. In addition, vetiver reduces stress and depression, according to studies. It also eases muscular pain and sprains and is a circulatory stimulant. For the complexion, it treats acne, wounds, and dry skin.

Wintergreen *Gaultheria procumbens*
The essential oil distilled from the leaves has a familiar, candylike, pick-me-up scent. It relieves muscular, nerve, and arthritic pain; irritation; psoriasis; and dandruff and softens skin. It is a common ingredient in herbal and drug-store liniments. Wintergreen essential oil is often Chinese wintergreen (*Gaultheria hookeri*) or birch (*Betula lenta*) tree bark, which contain the same compound, properties, and fragrance. *Note:* Wintergreen and birch essential oils are both toxic in large amounts, so use them carefully.

Ylang-Ylang *Cananga odorata*
These tropical flowers yield an intensely sweet, floral fragrance that is said to temper depression, anger, and frustration. It is also an aphrodisiac. A sedative, ylang-ylang in body oil reduces muscle spasms and blood pressure and helps with insomnia. As a hair tonic or in skin care products, it balances oil production so it is recommended mostly for dry skin and hair, but also for oily complexions. It is so sweet that high concentrations can actually produce headaches.

AROMATHERAPY
GLOSSARY

Absolute: This essential oil is extracted with a chemical solvent, which is then removed, leaving a pure essential oil. The process involves no heat, so it is used on plants like jasmine whose fragrance is destroyed by steam distillation's high heat. It can also be used to produce some expensive essential oils that can be distilled, such as rose. Some absolutes are so solid that they need to be warmed and thinned with alcohol. Some aromatherapists avoid using absolutes due to the toxicity of the solvent, even though it is removed to leave the pure essential oil.

Carbon dioxide extraction: CO_2 extraction uses high pressure without the high heat of distillation to create essential oils that usually carry a more complete fragrance that better matches the plant from which they originated. It is an expensive process that may become less so as demand for CO_2-extracted oils increases.

Carrier: Essential oils, to be used safely, almost always require dilution in some form of carrier, such as vegetable oil or alcohol.

Chemotype: This designates a plant that has a slightly different chemistry than others in the same species. They not only have a different fragrance, but their properties change along with the percentage of different compounds. These genetic variations typically occur when a plant grows in a different environment. Aromatherapists will seek out a certain chemotype because it is higher in a particular medicinal constituent.

Concrete: This is produced when a chemical solvent is used to dissolve the essential oils, as well as pigments and waxes, from a plant. The solvent is then removed through evaporation under pressure, leaving a sticky, soft wax that contains the essential oil.

Couperose skin: This sensitive type of skin that usually appears on the face is reddened and may show enlarged blood vessels. It is treated with gentle skin products.

Diffuser: This is a glass or ceramic apparatus that pumps a consistent fine mist of unheated fragrance to scent the air. It operates on an electric pump—find one that operates quietly. Thick oils such as vetiver, sandalwood, vanilla, myrrh need to be diluted with thinner essential oils with alcohol so they do not clog your diffuser. If it does get clogged, or if you want to get rid of a permeating scent, pour rubbing alcohol through it, then let the alcohol completely evaporate.

Distillation: Steam distillation extracts essential oils by passing steam through the plant matter to release the oil. The oil-laden steam is then forced into an enclosed condensation tube surrounded by a cold-water bath. The cold turns the steam back into water, separating out the oil.

Enfleurage: In this old method of extracting essential oils, the plant is placed on thin, warm layers of animal fat, which absorb the oil. Once the fat is saturated with fragrance, the oil is separated out. Rarely seen today, enfleurage was used for plants that are unable to withstand distillation's intense heat and have flowers that continue to produce essential oil after being picked, such as jasmine and tuberose.

Fixative: Most oils deteriorate with age, but fixative oils actually improve. They make the fragrance last in perfume and potpourri. Some fixative oils are clary sage, patchouli, sandalwood, vetiver, benzoin, frankincense, and myrrh.

Fixed oil: Vegetable oils are called fixed because their molecules are too large to escape naturally from the plant when it is heated or rubbed, as essential oils do. They are also not easily absorbed into the skin. Most vegetable oils are extracted by a combination of heat and pressure, although some, such as olive oil, can be cold pressed.

Fragrant or aromatherapy water: These waters are produced by adding essential oils to distilled water, generally ten to twelve drops per ounce. Due to their water content, they are moisturizing and hydrating. They are less effective, but also less expensive and easier to make, than hydrosols (see below) because you do not need a distiller to produce them. Spray or splash on a fragrant water after your shower, to cool down on a hot day, or to freshen your face.

GABA: Gamma-aminobutyric acid (GABA) is an amino acid that acts as a neurotransmitter to relax the nervous system and help regulate sleep, anxiety, and chronic pain by blocking impulses between nerve cells in the brain. Some essential oils promote GABA in the brain.

Herbal infusion: This is a fancy name for herb tea. When boiling water is poured over a fragrant herb to steep it, the essential oils extract into the water. Another type of herbal infusion submerges chopped, fragrant plants in warm vegetable oil to extract their oils. The essential oils migrate into the warm oil and the spent herbs are strained out.

Hydrosol: Steam distillation usually picks up the most water-soluble parts of essential oil. The oil is separated out, leaving this aromatic water, called a hydrosol. The hydrophilic compounds left in the water are good hydrating moisturizers for the complexion. Use them for facial sprays and room spritzers and to replace the water in aromatherapy formulas. They can also be used in foods and drinks safely. Turkish delight and the Indian lassi drink both contain the rose water hydrosol.

Volatile oil: Essential oils are also called volatile oils because they quickly evaporate into the air and dissipate.

MEASUREMENTS

The following chart will help you through the maze of measurements used in aromatherapy. It will guide you to finding the proper measurements when you convert formulas. Most books indicate formulas by the drop, but some use teaspoons or milliliters instead. The chart will also help you make price comparisons when you buy essential oils from different sources. This can get confusing because they are sold by the ounce, dram, or milliliter. The most common dilution for aromatherapy formulas is a 2 percent dilution, or twelve drops of essential oil per ounce of carrier (vegetable oil, alcohol, or water).

Approximate Measurement Conversion Chart

12.5 drops	⅛ tsp.	¹⁄₄₈ oz.	⅙ dram	⅝ mL
25 drops	¼ tsp.	¹⁄₂₄ oz.	⅓ dram	1¼ mL
100 drops	1 tsp.	¹⁄₁₆ oz.	1⅓ drams	5 mL
150 drops	1½ tsp.	¼ oz.	2 drams	7.4 mL
3 tsp.	1 tbsp.	½ oz.	4 drams	15 mL
24 tsp.	8 tbsp.	4 oz.	32 drams	118 mL
48 tsp.	16 tbsp.	8 oz.	64 drams	¼ L
96 tsp.	32 tbsp.	16 oz.	128 drams	½ L

RESOURCES

Educational Seminars and Products

American College of Healthcare Sciences

Dorene Petersen

PO Box 57

Lake Oswego, OR 97034

www.achs.edu

Correspondence course; seminars

American Herb Association

Kathi Keville

PO Box 2482

Nevada City, CA 95959

www.ahaherb.com

American Herb Association Quarterly Newsletter

Green Medicine Herb School seminars; essential oils; aroma-therapy products; aroma-herbalism tours to Tuscany

The Aromatherapy Course

Kurt Schnaubelt and Monica Hass

Original Swiss Aromatics

PO Box 66

San Rafael, CA 94903

www.pacificinstituteofaromatherapy.com

Correspondence course; seminars

Aura Cacia
Frontier Natural Products
PO Box 299
Norway, IA 52318
www.auracacia.com
Seminars; essential oils; aromatherapy products

The College of Botanical Healing Arts
Elizabeth Jones
PO Box 7542
Santa Cruz, CA 95061
www.cobha.org
Seminars; essential oils; aromatherapy products

White Lotus Aromatics
Christopher McMahon
602 S. Alder Street
Port Angeles, WA 98362
www.whitelotusaromatics.com
Essential oils; highly educational website

Organizations and Publications

Alliance of International Aromatherapists
www.alliance-aromatherapists.org
Membership journal

Aromatherapy Times
International Federation of Aromatherapists (UK)
www.ifaroma.org

Aromatherapy Today
www.aromatherapytoday.com

Canadian Federation of Aromatherapists
www.cfacanada.com
Membership newsletter

International Journal of Aromatherapy
www.sciencedirect.com/journal/
international-journal-of-aromatherapy

International Journal of Clinical Aromatherapy
www.ijca.net

National Association for Holistic Aromatherapy
www.naha.org
Membership journal

INDEX

Published in the United States by Ten Speed Press, an imprint of
Random House, a division of Penguin Random House LLC, New York.
www.tenspeed.com

Ten Speed Press and the Ten Speed Press colophon are registered
trademarks of Penguin Random House LLC.

Originally published in the United States and in different form as
Pocket Guide to Aromatherapy by Crossing Press, an imprint of
Random House, a division of Penguin Random House LLC, in 1996.

Library of Congress Cataloging-in-Publication Data
  Names: Keville, Kathi, author.
  Title: Pocket guide to essential oils / Kathi Keville.
  Description: [Revised edition]. | New York: Ten Speed Press, [2019]
    | Includes bibliographical references and index.
  Identifiers: LCCN 2019029974 | ISBN 9781984857828 (paperback) |
    ISBN 9781984857835 (epub)
  Subjects: LCSH: Aromatherapy.
  Classification: LCC RM666.A68 K483 2019 | DDC 615.3/219—dc23
    LC record available at https://lccn.loc.gov/2019029974

Trade Paperback ISBN: 978-1-9848-5782-8
eBook ISBN: 978-1-9848-5783-5

Printed in the United States of America

Design by Sarah Rose Weitzman

10 9 8 7 6 5 4 3 2

2020 Ten Speed Press Edition